T0246258

HOW K- DRAMAS CAN TRANSFORM YOUR LIFE

JEANIE Y. CHANG, LMFT

HOW

K- DRAMAS

CAN

TRANSFORM YOUR LIFE

POWERFUL LESSONS
ON BELONGINGNESS,
HEALING, AND
MENTAL HEALTH

WILEY

For general information on our other products and services or for technical support, please contact our Customer Care Department within the United States at (800) 762-2974, outside the United States at (317) 572-3993 or fax (317) 572-4002.

Wiley also publishes its books in a variety of electronic formats. Some content that appears in print may not be available in electronic formats. For more information about Wiley products, visit our web site at www.wiley.com.

Library of Congress Cataloging-in-Publication Data:

Names: Chang, Jeanie Y., author.
Title: How K-Dramas can transform your life : powerful lessons on belongingness, healing, and mental health / by Jeanie Y. Chang, LMFT.
Description: Hoboken, New Jersey : Wiley, [2024] | Includes bibliographical references and index.
Identifiers: LCCN 2023055086 (print) | LCCN 2023055087 (ebook) | ISBN 9781394210473 (hardback) | ISBN 9781394210497 (adobe pdf) | ISBN 9781394210480 (epub)
Subjects: LCSH: Mental health—Popular works. | Television programs—Korea (South)—Psychological aspects—Popular works. | Television plays, Korean—Psychological aspects—Popular works. | Television in counseling—Popular works. | Mental illness on television—Popular works. | Belonging (Social psychology)—Popular works.
Classification: LCC RA790.5 .C537 2024 (print) | LCC RA790.5 (ebook) | DDC 362.2095195—dc23/eng/20240125
LC record available at https://lccn.loc.gov/2023055086
LC ebook record available at https://lccn.loc.gov/2023055087

Cover Design: Paul McCarthy
Cover Image: © Getty Images | Flavio Coelho

SKY10069803_031524

This book is dedicated to all the K-Drama fans out there, validating why you love K-Dramas so much and giving you leverage to convince others to join our community.

I also dedicate this book to my younger sister, Kathy, who brought K-Dramas back into my life when I was on an unknowing hiatus.

And to my parents, Bae Sung Ho and Nam Kwang Hee, who instilled in me traditional Korean values that have rooted me in my identity today.

I'm also dedicating this book to my four kids, Melodie, Ian, Skyler, and Asher, because I'm so proud and thankful to be a mother, which is my main job!

Finally, this book is wholly dedicated to my super-supportive, patient husband of 26 years (as of this writing), who faithfully watches K-Dramas with me and enjoys hearing my deep dives while also giving me feedback. He has always been more excited about my success than I am.

Contents

Foreword

It has been remarkable witnessing the rise of K-Dramas as an international genre of storytelling. Since the pandemic, the popularity of shows and movies from Korea has been undeniable. What underlies that popularity is the way Koreans tell their stories. In the mix of love triangles and high school revenge, it is the way we as an audience are allowed to sit in the emotions of the characters that make us return to them. Korean dramas remind us about our stories, or rather, how we felt in our stories.

In talking about a particular K-Drama or specific moments in a K-Drama, we are able to slow-cook on those emotions and relate to them. That is how Jeanie Chang and I met. At a leadership conference of Korean Americans, we ended up sitting next to each other. Thus began a long and still ongoing conversation about our favorite K-Dramas and how they have helped the two of us on our storytelling journey.

Our most memorable discussion was caught live on the first presentation of Jeanie's Noona's Noonchi podcast. Of course, with Jeanie's superpower of listening, I opened myself to her about how K-Dramas helped me reconnect to my Korean heritage. We zeroed in on how K-Dramas help us find ourselves. Through my emotional connection with different storylines in Korean dramas, I learned to embrace my roots. As soon as I began to understand the wealth of stories from my homeland, I was able to fully understand how to tell my story. Leaning into K-Dramas and the complexities of my heritage helped me work with the Nickelodeon team to develop *Bossy Bear*. It also helped me understand how to tell my mother's story in my blog, *MommaKongSays*.

My conversations with Jeanie are always insightful, in part because we have the mutual language of K-Dramas, but mostly because Jeanie allows anyone to tap into their own inner drama. Much like the way Song Hye Kyo's character in *Descendants of the Sun* realizes that she is very much in love with her special forces lieutenant, or in *Thank You* when the grandmother character Kang Boo Ja quietly waves the little girl Bom (who has AIDS) to sit with her in her bathtub. Jeanie listens with the heart of a Korean drama producer. If you know those two specific show examples as I do, you'll recognize that K-Drama storytellers allow those looks of love and caution to replay over and over so that the viewer can see the impact of that moment from every angle and every character's perspective.

Jeanie allows you to express your *Jeong* and feel your *Han* by connecting you to similar moments in these dramas. She allows you to talk about them and see all the different ways to feel. In doing so, she is able to help you release subtle traumas by connecting you to something you have watched, by connecting you to something that allows you to feel despite the cultural and language barrier.

As you can see, I am a fan of Jeanie Chang! I know you will continue to find insights into yourselves through this book in the same way I do each moment I get to spend time with her. I look forward to more conversations with my friend and I cannot wait for you to read her book.

Chil Kong, Consulting Producer of Nickelodeon's
Bossy Bear and Adjunct Professor of Theater at
Bowie State University

Introduction

The Story of Noona's Noonchi

"K-Dramas saved me when I went through life traumas."

"K-Dramas helped heal my wounds."

"Through K-Dramas, I have found so many new friends from all over the world."

"K-Dramas make me feel less alone in this world."

This is a snapshot of what I hear from my clients and followers on a regular basis.

What if I told you Korean Dramas (K-Dramas) could also change the world? Maybe you're thinking, "Cool, tell me more because I love K-Dramas and want more validation to binge watch them." Or maybe you're saying to yourself, "You're kidding, right? How can a show like *Squid Game* change the world?" It's a bold statement, I know. That's what I'll be showing you throughout this book.

I'll start from the very beginning: with my own experience of K-Dramas both personally and as a Licensed Marriage and Family Therapist. K-Dramas have helped my mental health over the years, specifically with my cultural identity. What started out as self-care has blossomed into an integral part of my clinical work. I figured if they're helping me, they must be able to help others.

So I started talking about them in therapy sessions and in my virtual and in-person workshops. I'm not advocating for K-Dramas just because I enjoy them or because I'm Korean. My work as a licensed mental health professional trumps my cultural identity, and I'll always prioritize mental health and wellness. Having good mental health creates a ripple effect that leads to strong self-identity. And I believe K-Dramas can help.

The Noona's Noonchi channel started at the height of the pandemic, encouraged by college students who told me I should put all my content on YouTube. I found the thought funny. Me, start a YouTube channel? But it made sense because I had more content than I knew what to do with. I was also comfortable on camera. I started bringing K-Dramas consistently into my support groups, sessions, and talks early on in the pandemic because folks were so depressed and lonely that I needed something fun that would cheer them up in a unique way.

Of course, I had to think of a witty name. I knew right away I would use *noonchi* or *nunchi,* one of my favorite words in the Korean language. When I was a child, I received the highest compliment that a Korean adult can give: telling your parents (and you) that you have good noonchi. It's known as the Korean superpower, and I hold it near and dear to me because I am, after all, Korean.

The term refers to Korea's art of social and emotional intelligence. It's reading the room, gauging the context of people's reaction and the situations you're in, and assessing how you're feeling in reference to everything.

Koreans will tell you how complicated it is to explain noonchi. It's about being quick to act, think, and follow through in the most mature way possible. I use it daily and it's also an invaluable tool in my work, which is always client-facing. I became quite astute in using my noonchi virtually during the pandemic. In my line of work, I take my clients' or people's words with a grain of salt, even if they insist that they're feeling a certain way or doing fine or not doing fine. I have to dig deeper and use my noonchi to ask the questions that will get me answers so I can then help my clients, followers, and other people I deal with.

I wanted my YouTube channel and social media to be approachable, which is how I like to be in real life. "Noona" came to mind because it sounded witty next to noonchi. It means "big sister" in Korean, which is what boys call their older sisters or older girl friends. (In real life, I am actually an *unnie,* which means "older sister" or what women call their close older girlfriends, because I have a younger sister.) And so, Noona's Noonchi was born.

A Global K-Drama Community

"K-Dramas are for everyone."

I hear this often and it's important for me to point out that this point of view comes from non-Asians and non-Koreans. Gone are the days only Koreans and Asians watched K-Dramas. The Noona's Noonchi social media community is global. Today, most of my followers are from the United States, with the second biggest number from India. Based on my direct messages and interactions online, many of my U.S.-based followers are non-Asians—including white, Black, and Latinx—and only a fraction are Asian. I'm amazed at this wonderfully diverse community that has brought belongingness all over the world. It has positively impacted my mental health and gives profound meaning to my work.

In 2023, I launched Noona's Noonchi Tours, offering K-Cultural tours around South Korea, including popular K-Drama sites. My inaugural tours included only three Asian participants. I take this as a point of pride. It means I am being a good ambassador of my home country and influencing how my followers enjoy Korean culture through the eyes of their K-Drama experience. My tours are the first of their kind and I love bringing over people who are visiting Korea for the first time, eager to see the country depicted in their beloved K-Dramas, and, of course, who want to be closer to their beloved K-Pop artists.

Being in the social media influencer space, I have gotten to know other K-Culture influencers. The landscape is quite fascinating and worth exploring with you because it still blows me away. It's as global as you can get, which is something to write home about. There are quite a few prominent Korean and Korean American content creators and influencers, such as Priscilla Kwon (@priscillakwon) and Stephanie Kim (@tressuni), who cover K-Culture and cultural trends; Joanne Molinaro (@thekoreanvegan), as well as @maangchi and @koreanbapsang, who are popular for promoting Korean food; and Jane Park Kang (@janeparkang), who covers Korean culture in parenting and family. There are also well-known Korean content creators, like @mykoreandic, who address Korean culture, food, and trends, and @jfromkorea, who covers South Korea travel.

I've had the privilege of getting to know Jae Choi (@jfromkorea), who hosts tours around South Korea, along with his tour partner, @chrisbg, a Bulgarian content creator who lives in Korea. Chris helps run the ever-popular Instagram account @seoul.southkorea. The account has over a million followers and does a fantastic job of promoting Seoul and South Korea tourism. Chris says he believes South Korea travel is more popular than ever and that people are very eager to visit because they have the perception that it's the "Korean Dream."

This reminded me of growing up in an immigrant family and hearing so much about the "American Dream." To hear Chris talk about the "Korean Dream" just hit me emotionally. For people around the world to look at Korea like this is beautiful but surreal; it feels too good to be true. At the same time, I see what Chris is talking about because folks tell me, "Korea is on my bucket list." When I asked Jae why he thinks South Korea has become such a hot spot to visit, he took a moment to think about it and replied, "the Korean people." Jae acknowledges that

K-Content has played an important role, but in the end he believes the Korean people are what make Korea popular. On his travels, he's heard from many tourists about how they love seeing the Korean hospitality and the culture's emphasis on the collective and community. It's something I agree with, although I discuss in my mental health workshops that collectivism comes with its own stressors, like any cultural practice that has many nuances. Still, I believe the Korean people's collective mentality, a key aspect of Asian culture, is what has made Korea into a powerfully resilient global presence.

A testament of how global the K-Drama community has become is the number of social media accounts as well as influencers that are neither Korean nor Korean American. As far as I know, I'm the only Korean American influencer who covers the K-Drama niche and I stay as focused as I can on my mental health expertise. There are other Korean American and Asian American influencers out there who address Korean and Asian culture.

Amazingly, the social media influencer with the largest K-Drama community in the world is a young lady from Dubai. She's known as @deemalovesdrama on her socials, and she was the first-ever Noona's Noonchi Tours fellowship recipient who was provided the opportunity to attend my inaugural tour. With over 560,000 followers across Instagram, TikTok, and YouTube (at the time of this writing), Deema Abu Naser fell in love with K-Dramas when she was around 13 years old and started her account in 2019 because she loved the shows so much and wanted to find an outlet to talk about them. Deema shared on my inaugural tour how she feels such belonging with her K-Drama community and how that fuels her passion for being a content creator full time. I find it absolutely inspiring how a non-Korean and non-Asian built the largest K-Drama community in the world.

So much goes through my mind when I see non-Asians reviewing K-Dramas with such enthusiasm, as if I am unable to digest what's happening. These are folks who are publicly talking about K-Dramas and proud to be creating content about them. It wasn't too long ago that I could only mention K-Dramas with my husband and family because no one else would know what they were or didn't care to know. These influencers show just how appealing K-Dramas are on a global scale and that one can connect to them regardless of cultural descent.

Of course, many people still aren't aware that K-Dramas exist or don't seem to be interested in watching, and that is fine. The world is huge, and K-Dramas aren't for everyone. When I said this at a workshop in 2022, one woman in the audience responded, "Those folks don't know what they're missing!" Another one said, "They must be living under a rock if they don't know about K-Dramas."

There's an assumption that social media platforms, particularly TikTok, are exclusively for Gen Z. Being a Gen Xer, I used to think the same. However, I really liked what Priscilla Kwon shared about social media, which is largely influential in how K-Dramas have gone global and viral:

> You don't have to be young to enjoy social media. There's an audience for every single age group. For example, when *Squid Game* blew up, everyone was talking about it and there was such a fascination with it (across all ages). This made others who hadn't seen or heard of it want to jump on the bandwagon. That's what makes social media so powerful. You see and hear so many people talking about *Squid Game* that there's a fear of missing out (FOMO).

I know many folks my age and older who decided to become active on social media aside from Facebook and created Instagram and TikTok accounts because they wanted to follow K-Drama accounts, including myself, Deema, and others. They searched for K-Drama communities because they wanted to talk about their beloved shows. Social media is a huge reason why K-Dramas have boomed because they connect the community, and that FOMO promotes more K-Drama fans because the enthusiasm produces a ripple effect. Streaming services have also made K-Dramas go global because they're more accessible now than ever before. I used to downplay the impact of social media, but I can't deny that I've written this book and gained more speaking gigs thanks to my social media accounts.

It's one thing for me as a Korean American to find the K-Drama global effect surreal, but Korean nationals find it baffling. As a clinician and researcher at heart, I tend to ask Korean nationals I meet what they think about K-Dramas having such global appeal. Many question why foreigners enjoy K-Dramas so much and others find it downright amusing. I sometimes found myself trying to explain the global appeal of K-Dramas. I realized that most folks had never really thought about why they enjoy watching K-Dramas, but soon enough after thinking about it, they're able to answer. And it was like that with foreigners. Many Korean nationals indicated it was for entertainment purposes and a way to unwind after a long day. They saw it as a great form of escapism. Some say they like how K-Dramas portray certain issues that are occurring within Korean society, especially the recent dramas in the last few years, while others have said they enjoy watching with their families and their kids. Nevertheless, K-Dramas are a normal part of Korean society, as we would expect them to be, and their reasons for watching aren't too far off from ours.

JTBC (a South Korean TV network) producer director (PD) Christine Ko admits she was very surprised to hear such enthusiasm from K-Drama fans all over the world the several times she's been on the Clubhouse app. Christine says now that K-Content is so in demand, there's a much higher level of expectation in her work. It's a double-edged sword since it's an exciting time for K-Content. However, Christine is cautious about what kind of K-Dramas are being produced, since the industry has been asking these days, "What stories can we keep creating that are appealing to global audiences?" While I agreed with Christine that this is a thrilling time to be in the K-Content industry and there are stories to think about that can reach all audiences, I pleaded with her to stay grounded in Korean values, the good and bad of it all. My explanation to her on why K-Dramas have gained such traction is that the Korean culture and family values resonate with audiences in a time of adversity. Because people felt comforted watching K-Dramas, they grow more curious about the culture they're seeing. To stray from that would be a travesty. Christine agreed.

Why K-Dramas?

"I feel like my quality of life is pretty good when I'm watching two to three K-Dramas at a time, because it gets me excited."

– Korean American content creator, Priscilla Kwon.

K-Dramas are aspirational and inspirational. They allow us to strive, thrive, and hope for a better tomorrow. K-Dramas show us where we came from, who we are today, and what we could be. They're like a roadmap of life, guiding us in navigating life's speed bumps, roadblocks, twists, turns, dead ends, fork in the roads—you get my drift.

Joan MacDonald, a K-Content writer for *Forbes*, is someone I've long admired since I read all her articles. She says she feels K-Dramas are "so much more entertaining" than what she was watching on American TV. "In a very entertaining way, they deal with emotions and human relationships, and they feel very cathartic."

However, at its core, K-Dramas can change the world because they promote a beautiful experience of belongingness—a belongingness that the world needs now more than ever. In a post-pandemic world, belongingness inspires you to find yourself and build cross-racial and cross-cultural bridges. Belongingness with others across the globe makes the world feel smaller. Even though we may be across continents and oceans, K-Drama fans feel an undeniable closeness with one another because they share their love and enjoyment with others.

Belongingness is an innate human emotional need for survival. It's about being part of someone or something outside of yourself, just as critical as food, shelter, and water. It's guaranteed that when a K-Drama fan encounters another, the chemistry of belongingness happens.

Belongingness isn't just about kinship. It's also about connecting to yourself—your self-identity, values, and perspectives.

What K-Dramas do so well is developing their characters with such richness and depth. Shared experiences from trauma to achievements and successes all affect your emotional, social, and psychological well-being. Even if you tell me, "I'm a loner, I prefer being by myself," I'd tell you that your mental health will eventually take a hit since that leads to loneliness. "Loneliness kills," according to the longest-running study on happiness. Dr. Robert Waldinger, the Harvard psychiatrist leading the program, says, "Loneliness is as powerful as smoking or alcoholism."

K-Dramas reveal a spiderweb of complexities within us. The most obvious example is the K-Drama antagonist. While a character may start off being "bad," they may not necessarily end up that way by the end. It all becomes fuzzy once viewers begin to understand the backstory of the character as it's revealed. K-Dramas encourage viewers to develop empathy for characters outside of themselves and help them relate to experiences and emotions that aren't their own, a process called externalization, which I'll get into more detail later on. Compassion and empathy go hand in hand. Both are an essential element of belongingness.

People will tell you they love K-Dramas because of the storylines or the cute characters. But gaining insight into empathy and compassion—the core elements of the human existence, which weave into our mental health—is what really keeps us coming back to K-Dramas for more. Human beings are connective creatures, and what draws us to a K-Drama is its ability to help us evoke emotions in a less intimidating way, which in turn provides us an outlet or safe

space to process our thoughts and behaviors. Don't you think that the
world is a better place when we display more empathy and compassion for those around us, especially in a post-pandemic world? Priscilla Kwon called K-Dramas "a breath of fresh air" when the world
needed it the most. "I don't have this in my life and that's why it was
fun seeing it through K-Dramas."

My social media community really sparked me to dive into this
topic more deeply. One of my followers, Wayne Boatright, is a white
man in his sixties from the West Coast who spent seven years in prison
for a DUI that ended up killing someone. Wayne says he has accepted
the consequences, knowing a life was lost because of his actions, and
served his prison time with resolve and peace. Wayne says that in his
last few years in prison he bonded with his fellow inmates who introduced him to K-Dramas, and they would schedule time to watch
them together in the newsroom of the San Quentin jail where they
worked. In his own words:

> My saving grace in prison was finding K-Dramas on the back
> channels they have on prison television. Here we were as a larger
> group instead of in our own jail cells to experience K-Dramas
> together. I'm talking to these guys, all of whom were Black aside
> from me—we loved these K-Dramas and we felt connected.

Wayne says these were men who committed crimes like murder,
but their past crimes were irrelevant when it came time for K-Drama
watching. Each night, they eagerly sat together at 7 p.m. and experienced a belongingness that's indescribable in that San Quentin prison.
"We were transported to another world out of prison to another
place, another time, and it was enthralling."

His story moved me and still resonates today, perhaps because I
can imagine how difficult an environment like prison can be. Prison
inmates who have been sentenced for the most heinous crimes found
a belongingness in K-Dramas. Wayne pointed out that he was the

only white male in that institution, which we can imagine must make him feel vulnerable, but Wayne didn't indicate that to be the case at all except to say he felt part of a community of K-Drama fans, and that got him through the last few years of prison. To this day, Wayne is an avid K-Drama watcher who talks to me off and on about his favorites. I wouldn't have known about his poignant story had it not been for K-Dramas.

The K-Content Phenomenon

Do you know that 2021's *Squid Game* is Netflix's most-watched show in its history? This is an amazing statistic, along with the fact that 60% of Netflix subscribers have watched at least one Korean show. Netflix's co-CEO Ted Sarandos said himself that Korean content is proving to be the type of storytelling people want. Netflix has indicated it will invest $2.5 billion in South Korea over the next four years. (That gives me time to write a second book on K-Dramas for mental health!) Sarandos also says that one in five Netflix titles in Korea will come from a first-time writer or director because they believe success in Korea will lead to success globally.

The day that announcement came out, Korean Americans and K-Drama fans were texting one another in excitement. Disney+ also invested millions of dollars in producing Korean content. In fact, at the time of this writing, their 2023 K-Drama, *Moving* (a current favorite of mine), was its most popular show to date, which also happened to be the most expensive K-Drama production in history. Disney+ Korea wasn't doing well, but thanks to *Moving,* which also starred some of Korea's biggest stars, this all changed.

I believe these shows owe a lot to BTS and *Squid Game,* which catapulted Korean content onto a global scale. All BTS needs to do is mention what K-Drama they're watching or what their favorite Korean food is, and it'll be the next K-trend. *Squid Game* made history with its Emmy wins as Best Drama and Best Lead Actor

(Lee Jung Jae)—a first for a South Korean. When that happened, a wave of belongingness, or *Jeong*, rippled across the country. We felt that Jeong—the Korean concept for connection, kinship, affection—because we saw on a global scale, perhaps for the first time, that our culture was being hailed and centered. It's something many of us never expected to see.

Astonishing, considering where we were pre-pandemic, when I got scoffs for talking about K-Dramas in my work or was met with skepticism when I indicated K-Dramas can benefit your mental health. K-Dramas were fairly unknown to the general public until the pandemic. Joan MacDonald, prominent K-Content writer for *Forbes,* recalls that when she pitched stories on K-Content, she would be met with the response, "What does this have to do with our demographic?" Both Joan and I chuckled at how we're both living the global dream because she makes a living off writing about K-Content, which so many folks would love to do today.

Joan says her work stems from a passion she had for over 14 years when she first started watching K-Dramas. Back in 2012, Joan had only been watching K-Dramas for a couple of years, but knew she had to visit South Korea, which she did shortly after. The latest stat Joan says she knows of is how K-Drama viewership jumped by 200% in the United States amid the pandemic. Joan says, "These days K-Drama, K-Pop, K-Beauty is part of the younger folks' ordinary vocabulary." Joan says with a smile that the other day she was pleasantly surprised to hear her local Target playing BTS on the loudspeaker system. She couldn't have imagined that in 2014 when she first saw them perform. Neither could I.

When I first started listening to BTS back in 2015, no one had even heard of them. I really enjoyed their music early on. Now it seems I'm the one feeling skeptical when someone mentions the name of a K-Pop song or group that I've never heard of. I'm being schooled not only by other Asians, but white, Black, and Latinx people who look disappointed when I mention I haven't heard of who they are talking about. The same runs true when someone talks about K-Dramas they've watched, but I haven't.

A colleague had told me a couple summers ago that he wasn't sure that K-Dramas or even K-Pop would stay trending or even last. It was a passing comment, but it made me pause. But now, more than ever, K-Content is everywhere, on the major VOD, OTT platforms. Of course, there's Netflix, and popular Asian OTT Rakuten Viki and Kokowa, which only streams K-Content. There's even stiffer competition these days where we can watch our K-Content. It's a little overwhelming to have to choose from among so many platforms to figure out which K-Dramas I want to watch, because K-Dramas and other K-Content can now also be found on Disney+, Amazon Prime Video, Hulu, and Apple TV.

BTS members may be serving in the military now, but the group's impact is undeniable even when they're on a "break," per their 2022 announcement. The BTS Army is powerful. They're as loyal as they come. If any BTS member talks about the K-Drama they're watching, you bet Army will tune in, even if they were never K-Drama watchers. It's why I attribute the growth of K-Drama viewership to K-Pop fans. Many K-Drama fans indicate they started watching K-Dramas to see their favorite K-Pop artists who were acting in them. On the flip side, K-Drama lovers turned to K-Pop through the original soundtracks or music they heard in K-Dramas, as well as seeing their beloved K-Pop artists acting in the K-Dramas they were watching.

BTS has repeatedly broken records, and the influence of the Army is so strong, it can take over Twitter (X) feeds. In 2022, President Biden invited BTS to the White House to celebrate AANHPI Heritage Month and address anti-Asian hate. There's an iconic photo of BTS in the Oval Office and in the White House press room holding a press conference. That's an example of the incredible reach of K-Content. BTS was chosen to represent the AANHPI community amid a rise in anti-Asian hate.

The belongingness was three-fold. For Asians, it was seeing Asian representation at the White House. For BTS Army, it was a grandiose display of their beloved idol artists getting the recognition they deserved. For K-Drama fans and K-Pop stans, it was almost a rite of passage to see Korean celebrities front and center where they felt they belonged.

South Korean Tourism

Interest in South Korea and Korean culture—including tourism—has increased tremendously, thanks to K-Content. I still hear regularly "visiting S. Korea is top of my bucket list," and social media accounts that focus on South Korea tourism or influencer videos talking about South Korea travel tend to go viral. Thanks to K-Dramas and to K-Content overall, from films to webtoons, the South Korean tourism industry is enjoying a boom.

The Korea Tourism Organization (KTO) indicates the global influence of K-Content is "significantly influencing the inflow of foreign tourists to Korea." The KTO says the content they're watching on major OTT platforms such as Netflix, Disney+, Amazon Prime Video, and Apple TV has a direct correlation to this increase in tourism. According to the Korea Culture and Tourism Institute, most of the tourists visiting Korea in 2022 were from the United States, and the number of tourists from Southeast Asia surpassed those from China and Japan, which was a contrast from 2019, when most foreign tourists were from China and Japan. If the demand for my tours is any indication, I believe this number will only continue to grow.

K-Food

It's amazing how delicious the food looks in a K-Drama. It's one of the things the community bonds over while we watch. How we want to try the spicy rice cakes (tteokbokki), or eat ramen in a convenience store because the characters do that often. Korean food is being very much appreciated all over the world.

I have followers and clients who have asked me how I make my kimchi and what kind of *gochugaru* (Korean red pepper flakes) I use. I answer sheepishly that I don't know how to make kimchi, nor have I tried. Growing up, I was made fun of for having a "smelly" house because of the kimchi marinating in the fridge, so I internalized a sense of shame about kimchi and other strong-smelling Korean food. That's not why I don't make kimchi though. It's because my mother (umma) makes kimchi and I enjoy hers.

When others—especially non-Asians—tell me how much they love *doenjang jjigae* (fermented soybean paste soup), I'm amazed. It's one of the smelliest foods, and I struggle with it, my nose crinkling up when I see those special doenjang jars. I'm constantly working through healing from my experience of being ridiculed for eating Korean food.

Still, I feel giddy seeing that kimchi is recognized as one of the healthiest foods in the world with its probiotic benefits. In my workshops, I talk about kimchi and how it directly benefits mental health. There's a saying in the field of psychology that your gut is your second brain, so it's critical to take care of it with the right diet.

Some of the most popular social media sites and YouTube shows are non-Koreans enjoying Korean food or watching Koreans eat a huge amount of Korean food, which is called *mukbang*. Literally, all you're seeing is a Korean person eating, eating, and eating huge amounts of food

An integral part of my Meet You in Korea tour experience was the food, which is why picking out restaurants and menus was such a stressful but fun process. Trying Korean food for the first time, especially the street food and staple food dishes people see in the K-Dramas on a regular basis, was a big reason for the participants' eagerness to visit South Korea.

Korean food, rituals surrounding it, and how it's a tremendous part of the culture as seen in the K-Dramas is something people can easily glean from watching them. I have finally come to understand why my mother and my elders show such satisfaction and contentment when watching people eat their food. It's how I felt when I saw how happy my tour participants were trying all the new Korean food.

At a rest stop outside of Seoul, everyone was having a blast looking around the terrific food stands (Korea has amazing rest stops) and eagerly looked to me to talk about them so they could try them out. It was an "aha moment," realizing that this exuberant feeling is how my mom and Korean elders feel when they're serving food. Their fulfillment comes from folks looking happy and satisfied while eating. The tour folks weren't exactly eating something I prepared, but they were enjoying the food of my country of origin, and their happiness became my happiness.

How can the very food for which I was made fun of when growing up make people so happy now around the world? I get direct messages from followers showing off the fresh kimchi or kimchi stew they made. Folks take photos for me showing off the Korean food they're trying, whether they're in Korea or elsewhere in the world. The biggest comment I got for my inaugural tour was that they wanted to try more dishes seen in their beloved K-Dramas that weren't on the food tour itinerary. If that's the biggest critique about my tour, I'll take it. Food is at the core of Korean societal values and when I see it coveted globally, I cannot explain how much it means to me.

A Double-Edged Sword

Among the Korean American community and fellow Korean American influencers, there is a common sentiment. While it's nice getting this attention, which for the most part has been quite positive, it's not the attention we necessarily sought growing up. That seems to be the biggest misunderstanding. We just wanted the acknowledgment that we existed and belonged to be an active participant valued in American society. It's really that simple.

I'm sharing this because the global spotlight on Korean culture and content brings about a conflicted reaction at times. It's very much appreciated, but we're also protective of how our culture is represented, understood, and interpreted. Dabbling in the influencer space, I've spoken to other Korean American influencers who address this inner, and sometimes external, conflict when other social media influencers are speaking about Korean culture as if they're experts. Or if they're a K-Pop or K-Drama influencer, perhaps not quite getting the picture that being a K-Drama reviewer or K-Pop stan does not necessarily mean one understands what it's like being Korean.

While I'm here to write all about the benefits of K-Drama, it is nevertheless fictional, so the scenarios aren't necessarily reflective of Korean society. But their themes and messages sure are. Many times, when discussing Korean culture via a K-Drama, I make it clear that I haven't grown up living in Korean society. However, I do claim quite strongly my exposure to Korean culture growing up through my parents and extended family and I understand the cultural traditions and values because it's how I was raised.

The biggest pet peeve is when someone who is not of Korean descent tells us their opinions on Korean society and culture because they have a social media platform about Korean culture, or they've made a living in Korea. Max Harris Abrams, a Jewish American content creator living in Korea known as @Maxnotbeer, says he's mindful of this when he posts his content on TikTok and Instagram. He focuses on staying authentic and indicates he's the only one he shows on video. Max says he believes his content resonates with people because they're enjoying watching him explore Korean culture and food as if they're experiencing it all with him.

K Is for Korean: The Not-So-Soft Power

Attach a "K" before any word these days and you'll grab a stranger's attention and probably start an animated conversation. Maybe you mention it in front of someone you've known for a while and discover over the water cooler that you both love BTS. You start talking about becoming K-Drama lovers because BTS talks about them, and on you go, becoming fast friends, and the rest is history. Sound familiar?

Many once considered the Hallyu, or Korean Wave—the Chinese term referring to the tremendous growth of Korean pop culture—to be a mere trend. Hallyu is what they call an agent of "soft power," which has a cultural influence on society and economy. According to pop culture researchers, Hallyu 1.0 started with the boom of K-Dramas in the 1990s. Hallyu 2.0 followed with the rise of K-Pop. Hallyu 3.0 describes the K-Culture influence, with fascination for Korean language, K-Food, K-Beauty, and K-Trends. There's even a predicted Hallyu 4.0, which is also called "K-Style."

Korean culture goes deeper than any trend. I don't know if any of us predicted how Korea would hold such soft power and hard power. It was such a phenomenon to see how much Korean pop culture transformed Korea's economy, let alone the world. Korea was the little country in between two giant nations, and it had a history of standing helpless, particularly when looking at its record of Japanese colonization and Chinese influence.

This is both historically accurate and instrumental in describing my own identity formation. Korean wasn't anywhere near the forefront of people's minds. But then, as it built its soft power with such dynamic influence, Korea became a stronghold in between two former giants (China and Japan) and stood out on its own.

That's why seeing the fleeting term Hallyu brings out conflicting feelings in me. Coming from a mental health perspective, I feel that referring to the boom in Korean culture as Hallyu minimizes it into an unusual fad. For the sake of my mental health, why can't I choose to see that Korean culture blossomed on its own merits and became a natural part of societal growth? Through its turbulent history and fight for independence, Korea showed resilience to uphold its identity, putting itself on the global map and building its economy as a successful underdog.

In a mental health metaphor, I see Korea as a teenager at the center of a custody battle between two parents (Japan and China) going through a contentious divorce. Once the teen (Korea) turned 18 and had a chance to live on its own, it chose to make its own decisions, holding a cordial relationship with the parents, maintaining boundaries, and following its own path to reach success.

According to the Korea Economic Research Institute, Korea's economy grew by 37 trillion won or 29 billion U.S. dollars from 2017 to 2021, thanks particularly to Korean beauty products, K-Pop, and K-Content, which includes Korean Dramas and films.

I can't think of other words to describe a cultural phenomenon from a country like the word Hallyu. Folks may argue with me that it's a good thing to have Hallyu, that Korea's impact is so vast, there's a term for it. I'm concerned that using this term still "others" us.

Belongingness is about claiming and owning Korea's success as Koreans accomplished this on its own merits through blood, sweat, and tears. It's not an unusual phenomenon, a fleeting trend, or a passing fad. Korean culture is fully integrating into global systems because people love it.

There are dialectical forces happening at the same time, opposite elements that go hand in hand because we're complex. One example is how I feel happy about many people loving my Korean culture, but sad that it was rejected during my formative identity years. Excited that folks are talking about Korean culture from traditional media to social media, but nervous that they aren't getting their facts right and hoping that Korean culture won't be watered down, compromised, or culturally appropriated because everyone feels such belonging to the Korean culture.

That belongingness means that Korean is one of the fastest-growing languages in the world, outpacing its traditional rival, Chinese, in several markets. It is the seventh most studied language on the learning app Duolingo. That means it's the second-most-studied Asian language on the app. Research indicates more people are learning the Korean language thanks to the "Hallyu" wave and the rise in Korean content.

Many folks have shared with me that they hope to be able to watch K-Dramas without reading subtitles or be able to speak and understand when they travel to Korea. The keyword here is when, not if. This is the belongingness I'm talking about with the Korean culture, thanks to the beauty of Korean content and K-Pop. Watching K-Dramas, one cannot help getting immersed in the culture, and when that happens, you want to learn all you can about it.

Ironically, I grew up ashamed of the Korean language, and hearing it used to make me cringe. When I was seven years old, my mother told me I came home from school one day and declared I was not going to speak Korean at home, but only English from here on out. Honestly, I don't recall that moment, but I do remember thinking that I did not want to be Korean. My mother reminded me that I was beautifully bilingual until then. Part of me still holds some resentment against my parents for allowing me to just drop speaking Korean. But my mother told me I was so adamant about it at the time, and she and my father just wanted me to fit in at school.

We did end up speaking English at home, and that felt safe and comfortable. When I tell people that, they're astonished that we chose not to speak Korean. One of my father's goals was not to have a Korean accent. He wanted to assimilate, and not just survive, but thrive in American society. They already knew how to speak English when they came to the United States, but not to have a hint of a Korean accent seemed like an impressive feat, and my father accomplished it. A couple times in college he played a prank on me, calling me on the phone and pretending he was delivering pizza from Papa John's, and I didn't recognize him. In the Korean worldview, my father is a success, having graduated from the top university (Seoul National University) and graduating top two in his class for medical school. In fact, when I tell Koreans and Korean Americans my father graduated from Seoul National, there's an immediate respect for me just because I'm his daughter.

I'm talking about this because it's all part of my evolution in embracing my Koreanness. It is through years of watching K-Dramas that I have grown to appreciate my parents and the success they achieved even before coming to America. That's how powerful stories can be. K-Dramas tend to focus on the family, and seeing examples of different family systems and adult children interacting with their parents and children helped me better empathize with my own parents. One of my followers who is a white woman in her 50s told me that she was able to connect better with her mother-in-law thanks to K-Dramas. They helped her see things from her mother-in-law's point of view and she shares how they watch them together and talk about them.

A Black woman in her 50s who works in Washington, DC, tells me how her circle of friendships grew through watching K-Dramas. Like many others out here, she started watching at the height of the 2020 pandemic lockdown, beginning with *Crash Landing on You*, and the rest is history. "There were so many similarities between Korean culture and Black culture that I felt such a kinship." She continued, "I could relate to the trauma, family struggles, and feeling othered. I started opening myself up to Korean culture, even visiting Korea a few times, learning the language and making new Korean friends." I saw the joy in her eyes as she said how much K-Dramas have enhanced her life because of the other things that came with it.

What I marvel about this Black woman's experience is the depth of belongingness she feels to the Korean culture despite having just been introduced to it in 2020. She's fallen so hard for the Korean culture that she is completely in love.

When I traveled to South Korea last summer, she told me she felt so jealous. In fact, I heard that often from my clients and followers.

They would message me saying they wished they were in South Korea. I didn't even know how to respond. Perhaps because I spent so much of my childhood being jealous of everyone else and their cultures and race, I never thought that people would appreciate my own.

I still feel a giddiness whenever I hear from white folks, Black folks, and Latinx that they're learning Korean. They want to speak it out loud, they want to be fluent, they wished they could've learned the language sooner. Meanwhile, I tell them directly that they're probably more fluent than me at this point since I don't get the chance to practice Korean as much. It's funny when I see the looks I get sometimes, almost a disdain that I should be trying harder to speak Korean now. Times have changed, indeed.

If someone had told me years ago that this would be how I would celebrate my 50th year, I wouldn't have believed it. When I was growing up, I felt like a laughingstock because of my Koreanness, and there were many times when I would wish I could say I was just "American." Not Korean American, just American.

I remember feeling envious hearing others talking about their "all-American" families when we had Grandparents' Day at my school. I felt ashamed that I had to say that my grandparents couldn't make it because they lived in Korea. I remember feeling like an alien with my family in a country so distant that some people hadn't really thought about it.

I felt disconnected from my own culture, mainly because of my own parents' relationship to their cultural identity. I know that my parents must have struggled so much to maintain their sense of self that they held on to the Korea they knew in a country they didn't know and wanted their children (my sister and me) to hold on to it as well, even when we had no idea what that culture was. Writing this, I realize how far I've come in my identity journey, and how it has led me here, writing a book about K-Dramas for mental health.

This book deep dives into K-Dramas from a mental health perspective, but at the core of it all, I am talking about Korean culture—my culture and heritage. It's surreal to see how Korea is looked up to today. According to the *U.S. News & World Report* and Wharton School's Global Cultural Influence Rankings, South Korea's cultural influence rose to number seven in the world in 2022 from 31st in 2017, mainly due to Korean content such as *Squid Game* and BTS.

Our cultural identity powerfully intersects with mental health, and writing this book about Korea and Korean American culture makes my heart burst with pride. My hands are shaking as I write this. I know that many Korean Americans and Asian Americans can relate to what I'm sharing. Though we are still viewed as the perpetual foreigner, having this published by Wiley—a big publisher, no less—is a tremendous accomplishment, and oh so healing.

Growing up, I didn't imagine this kind of opportunity would ever come my way. If anything, I was usually on the defensive about my Korean culture, particularly the food and language. I recall often seeing condescending looks from people when they heard my mom's accent as if she was uneducated, even as the top graduate from a prestigious university in Korea. I wanted so badly for people to accept my culture and not insult it. It was hard to imagine that one day, Korean culture would be appreciated, and even celebrated.

I still do a double take when I see non-Koreans, and even non-Asians, making their own kimchi or sharing with me how they've graduated from beginner Korean language class to the intermediate level, or when someone wants to talk to me about a K-Drama they've watched that I haven't yet seen or even heard of. It feels good to see this much appreciation for my culture and feel like I belong for perhaps the first time in my life.

There's also some sadness with this, as I mentioned. It comes from wishing that this should've come sooner and how this could've been the reality all along. Dr. Josephine Kim, a senior lecturer on education at Harvard University said it so well: "I think about what it would've been like for those of us in our generation growing up in the United States to have had this during our formative developmental years and to be represented in such a way. To be looked at in an appreciative lens rather than be looked down upon."

She's around my age, and we both remember that in the 1980s and early 1990s, Korea and our culture didn't even cross people's minds. There were so many times that I wished I was Chinese or Japanese because that's what people assumed I was, and it felt embarrassing to say I was Korean. The look of confusion or even disdain was what I would tend to see. Some folks even asked, "What's that? Where is Korea?" I just wanted to crawl into the ground and disappear since that was easier than trying to explain about a country where I was born and having to defend my very existence. Considering it's my life's work now to address the intersectionality of mental health and Asian identity, I understand all too well how this feels and why it's distressing.

Dr. Kim closed her interview with me by saying, "I feel hopeful realizing that our children are growing up in this era where K-anything is looked upon so positively and favorably and what that means for their identity development. I feel all sorts of stuff!"

I do too, along with other complex emotions, which will be reflected in the next few chapters.

PART

I

The Powerful Intersectionality of K-Dramas and Mental Health

1

The Global Appeal of K-Dramas

"I stopped watching Western shows."

Belongingness for me is when I hear people say this, and how they'll choose Korean content any day of the week. I'll also hear that Western shows now feel like clickbait. My followers and friends often tell me how they can't watch anything else these days except K-Dramas because they find them wholesome, heartwarming, and "good for the soul," as content creator Priscilla Kwon would say.

Dr. David Tizzard, professor of Korean Studies at Seoul Women's University and Hanyang University, indicates Korean content is "unapologetically corny and they work because of it." He says, "Koreans lean into the cheesiness and that allows you to feel something. Korean dramas are designed to evoke emotion and a catharsis in the viewer. I consider myself a stoic man, a very masculine man, and I have been moved to tears on occasion because they do what they do."

All of the above, I believe, are benefiting their mental health, which is why I use K-Dramas in the first place. People tell me they love the family-friendly storylines and the emotional depth that comes from the characters and their growth. In essence, what people appreciate are the core values they see in K-Dramas. And that is why K-Drama viewership tripled in the pandemic. The pandemic was extremely stressful and folks needed comfort more than ever. They found it in K-Dramas, and once you watch one, people will tell you, it doesn't stop there.

We call it going down the rabbit hole, and you keep going down that rabbit hole. We all say it to each other very fondly, which further expands on the belongingness that K-Dramas promote. I have become the "popular girl in school," since people now crave everything about my Korean culture. They have told me they wished they were Korean, living in Korea, or married to a Korean. Suddenly I feel like I'm in the Twilight Zone because I'm among the cool crowd just because I am Korean. In my head I still find that quite surreal, considering that 35 years ago, being Korean was like being from another planet. The wistfulness of seeing how popular Korean culture is today is again where that sadness falls. Why couldn't all this come sooner so my mental health wasn't such a struggle growing up? It's just a fleeting question that arises every so often.

Let me go back to how folks love the fact that Korean content is easy on the eyes. For the most part, we don't have to worry about our parents, kids, or even grandparents walking in on a scene that's inappropriate due to graphic language, or cringe because of the sexually explicit scenes. That's what many people love about K-Dramas. They don't need to worry about constant violence, sex, or cussing in the scenes they watch. K-Dramas are comfortable, and this is important in terms of the impact on one's mental health. This is why many find K-Dramas a great form of self-care.

When you watch K-Dramas, the belongingness comes from immersing yourself in the experience of the characters and the stories surrounding them, which is why people end up falling in love with the Korean culture. After all, what we are seeing in K-Dramas reflects aspects of daily Korean life.

When you are so emotionally invested, how can you help but feel like you're getting to know another culture that you previously knew very little about? What I love about being part of the "in" crowd now is that it stems from love and belongingness.

It might seem that to be popular you have to be a "mean girl." You know that portrayal we see in American movies like Tina Fey's *Mean Girls*. While I did enjoy that movie, I'm glad that the popularity of Korean culture comes from the "nice" characters. People fall in love with the purity of the family-focused messages. Compared to many Western television shows and films, K-Dramas are refreshingly sweet and G or PG rated.

It's very important to recognize this as the root of how Korean culture gained its popularity. It is not rooted in toxicity. These Korean values felt like a perfect remedy during the Covid-19 lockdown when people around the world were feeling anxious, depressed, and traumatized in the middle of a historic global pandemic. While stuck at home, people craved comfort more than ever, and many told me they found solace in K-Dramas like *Crash Landing on You*. This K-Drama always seems to get mentioned as one of the shows that won folks over to the K-Drama genre.

Crash Landing on You became the gateway K-Drama, and suddenly, although I was already starting to use them to learn more about how they might help in mental health issues, they were proving to be an effective coping mechanism for health and healing during that difficult, uncertain time. Because many people are turning to K-Dramas now more than ever, I was encouraged to consider K-Dramas that would be a good starter show for those watching for the first time. There are iconic K-Dramas they must watch for the sake of understanding the K-Drama landscape and getting enough context about what K-Dramas are really about. So I've been recommending K-Dramas that I call rite-of-passage shows for rookie viewers.

When newer K-Drama watchers are asked about earlier K-Dramas (in the last 5 to 10 years) they might be met with a skeptical reaction of sorts, as if they're not really fans, because they aren't familiar with the earlier shows. It doesn't matter when you started watching K-Dramas, but as you delve deeper into the community, folks will bring up the iconic and older K-Dramas for reference, especially when speaking about their favorite actors. And the K-Dramas I recommend as a rite of passage also include those actors.

It's fascinating to see the trajectory of Korean societal themes, the actors' improvement, and how the behavior has shifted. For instance, many newer fans indicate they dislike the 2009 K-Drama *Boys Over Flowers* because they don't like the aggressive nature of the main lead. I don't disagree, but this K-Drama was a gateway for many, so it is iconic, as is the main character of Gu Jun Pyo.

I've heard that in Korea, Gu Jun Pyo's hairstyle was trending that year. The guide of my inaugural tour told me she recalls her son begging her to take him to the hair salon to get the Gu Jun Pyo look. I cracked up since it reminded me of women across America who wanted the Rachel hairdo from *Friends* back in 1995.

My Recommended Rite-of-Passage K-Dramas:

- *Goblin*
- *Boys Over Flowers*
- *Crash Landing on You*
- *Healer*
- *The Heirs*
- *What's Wrong with Secretary Kim*
- *Secret Garden*
- *My Love from the Star*
- *Coffee Prince*
- *Descendants of the Sun*
- *Mr. Sunshine*
- *Extraordinary Attorney Woo*
- *Itaewon Class*
- *Reply 1988*

Jeong = Noona's Noonchi Tours

Jeong is so important to me to talk about because that's also part of the global appeal of K-Dramas. I explained in the introduction this is the Korean concept of affection, kinship, connectedness, affinity, fondness; I could go on and on. Koreans know Jeong like the back of their hand but it's not as easy to explain in detail. However, Jeong is what I believe is the "it" factor that makes K-Dramas so special and appealing to all.

Angela Killoren, co-president of CJENM USA, agrees. "At the heart of K-Content is Jeong. It's literally this sense of connection, emotion, sincerity. All the different story points (in K-Dramas) happen around connection, whether it's lack or abundance or missing it, desiring for it. Jeong is the most universal truth."

Of course, I also believe Jeong is the most universal truth. The connection, the powerful belongingness is such an essential part of our existence. Jeong is what led me to create Noona's Noonchi Meet You in Korea Tours. At this point I've hosted two K-Drama- and K-Culture-oriented tours around South Korea for the public, particularly those who follow me on social media. K-Drama fans from around the world—most of whom who had never been to South Korea—traveled with me for eight days, visiting multiple cities where many K-Dramas were filmed, as well as seeing iconic and historic Korean cultural sites. Koreans in the tour industry have told me that what I created has never been done before. It's why it was one of the most challenging things I've ever done since I was trailblazing in this arena.

At one point I thought I wouldn't be able to do it because of all the logistics involved, and my time and resources were limited. However, as an extrovert I gain energy from interacting with others, and every time I conversed with my community I was reminded that this is a heart mission. Creating these K-Drama tours, where my team and I started from scratch with the itinerary, is rooted in Jeong: the Jeong for my community, the Jeong for my heritage, the Jeong for my culture. Jeong is that kinship my Noona's Noonchi community feels with South Korean culture, which is why my two inaugural tours sold out in less than two weeks. People felt like they were familiar with the culture, and I loved seeing their faces when they recognized the food and the places, and observed the people. Seeing my heritage through the eyes of my followers was unforgettable. The thrill in their voices made up for years of angst I went through hiding my culture and wishing I was anything but Korean.

Here is what I heard from the inaugural September tour participants. When I'm feeling down or the going gets tough, I'll just read these comments and be reminded of why I do what I do:

> "This tour truly captured lightning in a bottle with the fantastic chemistry of the participants and the organizers. I felt that there was so much for us to see and do while also giving space for some free time to explore. Watching dramas since my return has added an extra element of the 'I've been there' feeling, and I love it. This tour was the perfect balance of examining why K-Drama is so beneficial for mental health while also exploring the culture and history of an amazing country."

> "I have not felt this physically, mentally, and emotionally healthy for a long time. This trip was the key to that feeling! Thank you for all that you did and for organizing such a wonderful experience."

> "Thank you for this tour. Thanks to this experience, I see the world in a different perspective. It feels like a dream. Thank you, Jeanie, and all the team!"

> "Thank you for making this dream come true indeed, Jeanie! This was one of the best experiences of my life! You and your tour team went above and beyond for us and created an incredible tour from start to end. I miss everything and everyone already! Can't believe this happened and can't wait to do the reunion trip."

Many of the tour folks shared that they didn't really have people to talk with about K-Dramas and are so thankful for this community. Deema has said it's the camaraderie she has with her followers and the rewarding feeling of building a vastly engaged K-Drama community that has enhanced her well-being. What started as a lonely road is now a friendship-filled freeway of endless conversations about K-Dramas. This was the common denominator of my inaugural tour. It's why folks were able to become fast friends and avoid having to go through the awkward small talk. They came to the Noona's Noonchi Meet You in Korea Tour because they love K-Dramas, and therefore couldn't wait to experience the Korean culture they grew to love and visit a country they came to know. It felt like a dream to be walking with my very first tour group as we followed my tour guide to our dinner location.

Nineteen participants had flown to South Korea, thrilled to be on a tour of my country of origin to experience in real life the culture and people they came to love through K-Dramas. After some time, one of them, a South African American woman, turned to me and said, "I've only been here a day and a half, and I feel like I belong here. Strangely, this feels like home, and I want to find a way to live here." My response: "Really?! Are you serious?"

No matter how much I knew that these folks had anticipated this tour, it still amazed me how immediate the connection was for her. I admitted to her that I didn't expect the statement to come from her at all, as a South African American woman. She agreed that it sounded far-fetched, but there was no denying how she felt. Throughout the tour, she started researching ways to work and live in Seoul. To this day, it's a goal that she is willing to work toward.

One of the things she shared with me when she got back to the United States after flying home with a fellow participant was how they were both whining about being back home and pining for South Korea. Her words brought out such emotions in me: I didn't expect these folks to truly love being in South Korea, and I was just beginning to absorb the impact of what I had created in Noona's Noonchi Tours. Again I was reminded that all of this, including the dream tour, wouldn't have happened without my passion for K-Dramas and sharing this with a growing community.

K-Drama Characters

People have also told me how much they appreciate the character development in K-Dramas, and I believe the complexity mimics real life. A theory in psychology holds that black-and-white thinking isn't productive, especially when it comes to depression. Western TV shows tend to have such clear-cut portrayals; for example, we generally see a clear antagonist and protagonist, good versus evil. Real life doesn't work that way, as I tell my clients. There are many grays in life, in decision-making, and yes, even in people.

In the field of psychology, dialectics refers to polar opposite elements that can exist hand in hand, such as love and hate, or peace and war. I talk about dialectics quite a bit in my work because that's what conflict looks like. You want to change, but it's so hard to change because the first response to change is resistance. A good example of a dialectic on the personal front is my own experience as a Korean American. I love being Korean, but there are things about Korean culture that I still struggle with. For instance, I dislike the patriarchal tendencies and the intensity of the stress surrounding education, but in the same breath, I appreciate Korea's traditional family values, and the emphasis on education is why I believe I have a high threshold for stress and anxiety, which aid my work as a clinician. That's all thanks to my parents, who pushed me quite hard while I was growing up, even though it felt terrible at the time. That is a dialectic to which I find many immigrant children can relate.

Dialectics correlate to K-Drama characters through mental health, particularly their emotional well-being. In K-Dramas, we see characters experience a plethora of emotions displaying the dialectics I'm speaking about. Dialectical Behavioral Therapy (DBT) is one of the psychotherapy modalities I use often in my work. DBT is a newer modality that was developed in the 1970s by psychologist Marsha Linehan, who was struggling with her own mental illness. DBT combines Cognitive Behavioral Therapy (CBT) and humanism with the concept of dialectics. It is the first psychotherapy to incorporate the practice of mindfulness, which is why I use it in my work, because I am trained in mindfulness-based stress reduction and recommend all my clients practice mindfulness. I was once the biggest skeptic on mindfulness, but once I started incorporating it in what I call daily mental health hygiene, I realized how impactful and effective it could be. I talk often about how K-Dramas help us practice mindfulness because we are engrossed in the story and focused on the here and now; even if it's an imagined story, it is still mindfulness. Those who depend on the subtitles indicate they have little choice but to concentrate on what's being said by reading them and cannot do anything, so they end up feeling like they've rested. It's why I say K-Dramas are a good balance of realism and escapism.

K-Dramas are popular because of the tropes. I know you're probably thinking, "No, I dislike the tropes, thank you very much, because they're so predictable." However, we actually lean on the tropes whether we know and appreciate it or not. As K-Drama fans will tell you, the tropes are easily identifiable. The predictability is exactly what makes K-Dramas so appealing. K-Dramas have a formula to them. They tend to be one season of 12 to 20 episodes (though more K-Dramas are doing second seasons), and they almost always have happy endings.

The happy ending trope is one of the main reasons why people enjoy K-Dramas so much, though they may not admit it. But then there's that K-Drama with a sad ending. Spoiler alert: the ending of the 2022 *Twenty-Five Twenty-One* K-Drama had so many viewers up in arms, particularly the Gen Z population. The ending wasn't sad, but it wasn't the happily-ever-after that K-Dramas tend to have, and I still hear from folks who were quite upset by it. The not-so-happy ending left people in despair; some even said they felt "traumatized." As a therapist, I don't discount their feelings, since that was their experience.

We need the tropes because, as research indicates, predictability is helpful in preventing trauma and managing distress. It's why I indicate the importance of maintaining a routine or schedule to keep a semblance of control. K-Drama tropes, which is a large part of their formula storytelling, provide stress management because folks feel in control of what they're watching. Based on my own research and K-Drama ratings we see from South Korea, the most popular, talked-about K-Dramas are those that contain the classic tropes, including the happy ending, the love triangle, the rich man (the *chaebol* in Korean) falling in love with the woman from a poor family, best friends to lovers or enemies to lovers, and the toxic workplace or family.

As I write, the most talked about K-Drama in Korea and globally is *King the Land*. It is chockfull of all the romantic tropes—including the chaebol, heir to a large hotel conglomerate—falling in love with an ordinary hotel worker, and K-Drama fans are buzzing over it, including the ever-predictable kiss that tends to occur in episode eight, according to the K-Drama formula. These tropes help us feel grounded, rooted in what we find to be comfortable, and help keep us at ease.

2

K-Dramas Are for Self-Care

Yes, K–Dramas really are for self-care. They have been a source of comfort for viewers for many years, whether they realize it or not. Watching K–Dramas helped me pivot my career when I was unhappy and unfulfilled, encouraging me to follow the path to what I am doing now. K–Dramas are how I unwind, decompress, spend quality time with my husband (and sometimes my kids), all with reflection and an introspective mind. They have become the default, most accessible self-care for many of my clients and followers.

Noona's Noonchi started because K–Dramas helped me, so I figured they would help others too. I've also found that K–Dramas are a source of comfort for Korean nationals. You might think this was the case each time, but how K–Dramas are received by Koreans is quite different in the sense that they haven't been too keen on its connection to their well-being. They're more motivated by the fact that it brings them pure entertainment, showing off their favorite actors and displaying societal themes they relate to.

In a sense, I have had to work hard to explain the connection between mental health and Korea's beloved K–Dramas to Koreans. For instance, I have heard from folks my age as well as people from the MZ Generation (a term used only in South Korea to refer collectively to both Millennials and Gen Z) that when *Misaeng* (a popular office K–Drama) came out in 2014, Korean males cried while watching it. Women have told me they saw their husbands and fathers expressing emotions perhaps for the first time while *Misaeng* was showing because they felt so validated seeing their own work life or office experience being portrayed in that K–Drama.

How wonderful to hear how a K–Drama made them felt seen and heard, perhaps for the first time in their career, or even their lives. These men cried because they had been struggling internally, feeling alone in their work experiences while balancing the pressures of family and society. When they saw their own lives represented in *Misaeng*, I believe the tears came because it was a relief to finally express their pent-up emotions. Hearing about this (which was fairly recent, due

17

to my research for this book) made me realize as a clinician that using K-Dramas for mental health is just as significant, if not more so, in South Korea. Koreans just don't realize it quite yet because mental health and the field of psychology is lagging in the country, for now. However, it will soon catch up.

I believe K-Dramas and mental health have a powerful intersectionality. I wouldn't be writing this book today if others didn't believe there was a direct correlation as well. As I mentioned earlier, I figured they were helping me, so they must be able to help others. When you're inspired by something or someone, you have the desire to inspire, so you want to share that experience with others. I enjoyed watching K-Dramas so much because they made me feel good and I wanted to share in that experience with others. That belongingness I find is true for others who have realized what K-Dramas have done in their lives.

I have a trademarked mental health framework called Cultural Confidence®, which I correlate to K-Dramas for mental health. Cultural Confidence®, outlines four elements that I find the most in my work, including mental health, identity, mindfulness, and resilience. Of course, all four of these elements are threaded throughout K-Dramas, which is why I use them in my work. Pre-pandemic, though K-Dramas were quite popular, they weren't as global as they are now, so when I talked about how K-Dramas can benefit your mental health, I noticed people's opinions of me shifted, and not in a positive way. I was often met with skepticism or would get a chuckle here and there when I talked about how K-Dramas could be useful. Obviously I have become much bolder, thanks to *Squid Game* putting them on the map. Now I tell folks that K-Dramas can change your life for the better. They can transform you, help you make meaning in your life, provide coping skills, and increase mindfulness practice. What they do so well is stimulate an expression of emotion, but it is not meant to replace therapy. K-Dramas are not therapy (coming from a therapist), but there are so many things that are therapeutic about them, especially when it comes to understanding your emotions. It's why I indicate a "dose" of a K-Drama a day can be beneficial; I'm not advocating binge-watching K-Dramas all day so that you neglect your responsibilities. I also don't like the term "K-Drama therapy," even though that phrase appears many times, whether it's in articles in which I am interviewed or all over social media.

I watch K-Dramas for my own self-care. It all began in 1992 when I spent the summer at Yonsei University in Seoul to attend a summer language program for Korean Americans. This was the summer I realized that being Korean wasn't so bad after all. As I've mentioned before, I had little interest in learning about my Korean heritage when I was growing up. The culture was forced upon me by my parents, who seemed to be stuck in 1974 Korea and parented me that way. I knew they were doing their best with what they knew. I felt strong resentment toward Korea and all things Korean until that pivotal summer in 1992.

When I was in Korea that year and watched the K-Drama *Jealousy* (called *Jil-tu* in Korean), it stopped me in my tracks. It showed me that the lead actress—who was very popular at the time—was someone I liked for who she was and what she looked like. For the first time, I started thinking that being Korean like her wasn't a bad thing. She was cute and spunky, and the leading man was good-looking. And this K-Drama had the classic best-friends-to-lovers trope.

Aside from Korean language and culture school for four hours a day, I spent the rest of the time with fellow Korean Americans from all over the United States. The belongingness of having people who share the same identity and similar experiences took me down a path of poignant self-discovery to open myself up to my culture. It took 18 years. That K-Drama, *Jealousy,* was just the beginning of tumbling happily down the rabbit hole and thus beginning my love for K-Dramas.

I tell people fondly that well before streaming services we relied on VHS tapes. We would have to go to the local Korean market to rent

K-Dramas on VHS and had two to three days to watch them before we had to return them. Binging was necessary back then because we had a time limit, and this made K-Dramas even more coveted. I was gobbling it all up. I remember falling in love like the female leads were and enjoying seeing everyday Korean culture. Although I was using the subtitles, I liked improving my Korean by hearing the language often. Then as now, K-Dramas told fabulous stories. In the early 1990s through the early 2000s, through K-Dramas I was experiencing my culture in a way that was unique. I fell in love with myself, my culture, my heritage, my background, my everything because I appreciated how happy K-Dramas made me feel. I was lucky because after I got married in 1998, my husband (who's also Korean American) enjoyed them with me. I've been watching K-Dramas now for 32 years, if you do the math right, with a multiyear hiatus due to the busyness of raising four kids born within six years.

Those who enjoy K-Dramas can tell you how much they like them and even how good they make them feel. However, folks struggle with telling you why K-dramas make them feel the way they do. I realize now that my K-Drama watching experience, beginning from 1992 when I was 18 years old and over the years, was positioning me to do what I am doing today. My work in mental health is technically my third career. What I appreciate is that unbeknownst to me, I was getting K-Drama watching experience under my belt to build the credibility in my work today. I'm not talking about being a K-Drama veteran. I am talking about how many years I have had watching K-Dramas that have benefited my mental health to give me the authenticity for the authority I need to help my clients and colleagues. At the end of the day, I need to practice what I teach to be impactful and effective. I need to know what I am talking about and be able to answer questions when needed. The truth is that K-Dramas are a significant part of my daily life, my self-care, my identity formation, and my confidence, and they educate me more about me. I have gotten proficient at defending my case when needed because for 32 years, K–Dramas have meant so much for my emotional, social, and psychological well-being.

> "Look at where K–Dramas are now, so proud of the work you're doing!"

My good friend from childhood who's known me since I was in elementary school recently sent this public message to me on Facebook. Although you all may assume she's giving me well wishes because I'm using K–Dramas in my work, there's so much more meaning to this.

I grew up in a tight-knit Korean American church and my youth group was super close. There were around 10 of us and I think back so fondly on those days when we were discovering our Korean American identity together. This co-ed group was around the same age, and after our first year of college, we came back together over winter break obsessed (okay, some less than others) over K–Dramas. This was after I fell in love with the 1992 K–Drama *Jealousy* and was enthralled with everything Korean because I had never bothered to learn about my culture until then. When we got together, we videotaped ourselves acting out the iconic introduction to *Jealousy*, with the music and everything. I'm chuckling as I write this because it's bringing back such wonderful memories. What nostalgia. To see where things are now as I write this book is very emotional. My childhood pals and I also videotaped us acting out scenes from *Sandglass*, a very famous 1995 K–Drama where Lee Jung Jae of *Squid Game* fame had his breakout role as the beloved bodyguard of the female heroine. We have these makeshift K–Drama videos all on VHS tapes safely stored away at my friend's house. Oh, how much I would give to see them now.

Our group of pals got even closer during this time as we were "filming," re-creating the K–Dramas we were enjoying. Back then in the 1990s, barely anyone outside of the Korean and Korean American community even knew about K-Dramas, let alone being interested in them. This was our own private, sacred world where we felt safe and could relish our Korean culture together as friends. I didn't realize that at the time, my mental health, with which I had struggled on my own due to intense internal cultural conflict, was being improved through these K-Drama reenactments with my peers. There was a keen understanding among us that we knew what these K-Dramas meant and how well they provided us the representation we so badly needed but never got throughout our childhood and teen years.

Nevertheless, these OG K-Dramas came at a time when we were just starting college, which I think couldn't have been better timing. The Jeong among us, the enjoyment in the K-Drama characters and stories boosted my self-confidence at the time, and this in turn boosted my mental health. I know my childhood pals are shaking their heads in a good way, surprised but not surprised, that I am making a living talking about these K-Dramas now. I recall how much fun it was pretending to be these K-Drama characters and talking about the culture in such a wonderful way that we hadn't been doing until that point. It'll always be a special time when K-Dramas were unknown, but we found them to be gold mines for ourselves. We discovered gold because I know for all of us moving forward, we better defined who we were as Korean Americans and felt pride surrounding our Korean heritage, perhaps for the first time as college kids.

Marriage and Family

K-Dramas are also good for my marriage and family. They have enhanced my marriage of 26 years because my husband also enjoys watching them. Lucky me. As one who has treated couples, I can tell you that it is very important for a relationship where couples can enjoy an activity or experience together. I feel blessed that my husband is just as enthusiastic about K-Dramas as I am. He was raised in Korea until the age of 10 and then immigrated to Los Angeles, so he grew up more in tune with Korean culture than I did. In fact, my husband watches more K-Dramas than I do. He's less picky than I am when it comes to genres and will watch them all if they're interesting to him, whereas I cannot watch dark K-Dramas that focus on evil spirits or psychopaths, perhaps because it hits too close to home in my line of work. My husband is my best K-Drama watching partner and he also sees their value, particularly in our marriage and family. We'll watch them together and discuss scenes or quotes that have an impact on us or our parenting. We learn from what we watch and apply it in our lives. But K-Dramas are most beneficial for our marriage because they bring us closer together physically, both literally and in our love life. K-Dramas almost always feature a love story that's as cheesy (as Dr. Tizzard pointed out) and cringy (as my kids would say) as it gets. However, this is the type of cringy that puts a smile on your face and gives you the warm fuzzies because it's that romantic. It makes you want to cuddle and spoon with your significant other. When watching love scenes (in K-Dramas, they're generally rated G or PG), the love, bonding hormone, oxytocin, is released, so it adds to the appeal. It's also why K-Drama "homework" can be helpful to incorporate when working with couples.

Reply 1988, *2015*

Our family is better off because of K-Dramas. Our family K-Drama is *Reply 1988*. We love it, our kids love it. We watched it together. Our 19-year-old son even wrote about this show for his college essay. He talked about how he got to know his maternal grandparents, my parents, by watching *Reply 1988* with them. I didn't know this until I read his essay, but he shared how my father talked about feeling nostalgic when they watched it. They didn't live in Korea in the 1980s, having immigrated to the United States in 1974 when I was a baby, so they told my son they got to experience the Korea they missed by watching *Reply 1988*. That was very touching, and I had no idea they felt such a loss. That was their way of sharing their grief with my son.

My son talked about experiencing Jeong through this K-Drama, which motivated him to write about it in his college essay.

Reply 1988 also helped me understand myself as an older sister, many years later. Just a few years ago over Thanksgiving break, my sister told me, while we were watching *Reply 1988* together for the umpteenth time, that I am Bora. If you've watched the show, you know exactly the prickly, angry type of sister she is. She was harsh and mean to her younger siblings, particularly Deok Sun, her younger sister, who's the female protagonist of the K-Drama.

I was quite offended when my sister told me I was Bora. My parents were there when she said it, and they cracked up. They didn't disagree, so they weren't going to defend me in that moment. I was indignant. From a noonchi perspective, I knew she hit a nerve because I was defensive. We kept watching, and I was going to argue her point when I saw a family scene that reminded me of how I was when I was younger. Bora tried to sneak into the house after a day of protesting, which her parents didn't want her to do. *Reply 1988* was set during a period of history where the government was in turmoil and students were leading protests. When Bora's father caught her, he got angry and forbid her from going out again to protest, but Bora defiantly responded that she would continue protesting if she wanted to.

I'm not sure why I didn't make the connection before, but that's exactly how I behaved with my parents in front of my sister. In that moment of openness and then acceptance, I realized that I could see how I was like Bora to my sister. It's not like I remember those exact moments I was mean to her, but I do recall resenting how much pressure I felt as an older sister and couldn't get away with anything, while it looked like she was getting off easy. I was jealous of her being the younger sister. I was also letting off steam due to my own teenage angst and the stress of my parents' expectations, and my sister was an easy target. It is very different now though; the age gap doesn't feel as big as it used to, and we are now more like friends.

People can be mean when they're feeling hurt or frustrated with themselves. They tend to lash out at those around them or the people they are either jealous or resentful of. Hence, my own conclusion that my sister made sense, as hard and humbling it was to accept. I was the loudest one in the family during my teenage years (as Bora was) and didn't quite know how to communicate with my parents as my sister may have done. As I pondered the correlation between myself and Bora, I also had a revelation that Bora's awkwardness with both her parents, especially her father, was so much like my own situation. We see her calm, cool, and collected around her parents; though she expressed some emotions through her words, she held it together. It wasn't until her wedding day that the dam of emotion burst wide open, and her tears fell like a waterfall, as did mine when watching that scene.

My Favorite Family-Focused K-Dramas
- *The Good Bad Mother*
- *My Daughter, Seoyoung*
- *Go Back Couple*
- *Reply Series (1997, 1996, 1988)*
- *Our Blues*
- *My Father Is Strange*
- *One Spring Night*
- *My Liberation Notes*
- *Once Again*
- *My Unfamiliar Family*

Intergenerationality

Of course, it isn't only our family. K-Dramas can bring families closer together because they're family-oriented, as is the Korean (and Asian) culture. Clients and followers have told me they have grown to better understand their families, particularly their parents and what makes them tick. This runs true for both Asian and non-Asian families. This is how I began using K-Dramas in the first place, to help clients improve family dynamics, increase communication, and manage conflict. There's a term for this: intergenerationality, which refers to the relational dynamics between members of different generations. What I love hearing from clients is how, when watching K-Dramas with their parents, they were able to pause a scene and share with their parents that they had to point something out to them. For instance, I had a client indicate to her mother that she cannot really have a conversation with her because her mother either dismisses what she shares or speaks condescendingly to her. The client had experienced a heartbreaking breakup with her fiancé and her mother insisted it was her own fault. This was extremely hurtful for the client, who wanted to mourn in peace but hoped her mother would be supportive. According to the client, her mother wasn't really giving the client a safe space to share her pain by dismissing her when she tried to share or spoke condescendingly to her.

Dear My Friends, *2017*

It wasn't until they were watching a tumultuous scene between mother and daughter in *Dear My Friends*, a 2017 K-Drama, that they had a breakthrough. The client told me she paused the scene and felt empowered to tell her right then and there that she also wanted to throw a glass vase across the room like the daughter in the drama because she was that angry with her mother. It stunned the mother because the scene in *Dear My Friends* was emotionally charged, but she was able to connect the dots between what they saw in the K-Drama when it came to mother-daughter dynamics to their own relationship where they were always disengaged and noncommunicative. It was at the breaking point, just like they saw in the *Dear My Friends* where the daughter couldn't take it anymore. In this case, I was able to help begin mending a mother-daughter relationship following a K-Drama watching experience. The client had been struggling with breaking through to her mother and a K-Drama helped her do it.

Incidentally, I didn't suggest the K-Drama to this client; she watched it of her own accord. However, after this case, it has been one of the K-Dramas I recommend to clients to understand the aging population that doesn't get the attention it deserves, especially now more than ever as I am seeing more news stories about them being neglected. *Dear My Friends* humanizes our aging parents and their conflicts. With their core value of wisdom and leaving a legacy based on Erik Erikson's eighth stage of psychosocial development, they are set in their ways. They can labor to communicate their needs and struggles because they were the ones caring for others. *Dear My Friends* also showed a character exhibiting early signs of dementia, which was a personal experience of mine with my maternal grandmother and for many others as well. There are poignant scenes where the characters ask each other who is wearing adult diapers. They laughed about it rather than being ashamed, and I thought that was a terrific portrayal for us viewers to see. Again, it's to bring about an understanding of intergenerationality and how powerful of a role it plays in our overall system of support.

It's important to keep in mind that intergenerationality does not just necessarily apply to families. It refers to all relationships and interactions among and between different generations. Many K-Dramas showcase this as well since K-Dramas are community-centric. For example, we see positive and healthy examples of nonfamily intergenerationality in K-Dramas, such as *When the Camellia Blooms*, where the female protagonist Dong Baek, a single mother of a middle school son, has a close relationship with her boyfriend's mother. The boyfriend's mother also grows close to Dong Baek's son, taking the role of his paternal grandmother (*halmuni*) even though they aren't blood relations.

K-Dramas Showing the Healing Power of Intergenerational Relationships:

- *Navillera*
- *Mr. Sunshine*
- *My Mister*
- *Our Blues*
- *Hometown Cha-Cha-Cha*

Healthy Emotionality

There's a beautiful line in episode 12 of *Be Melodramatic*. I often use this K-Drama when explaining the healthiness of emotional expression. In its English translation, the line goes something like this: "Tears kept in your heart can become an illness, while tears that are let go will evaporate and disappear in this world." That is a great way to explain why a crucial aspect of mental health is to release and express one's emotions when needed and when we are ready.

Forbes writer Joan MacDonald says that when watching K-Dramas she enjoys the release because "sometimes you need to feel things." Joan says there are times when you need to feel anger and sorrow, and understand what it feels like to be wronged. "When someone is a villain in a K-Drama, you just hate them and that's somehow cathartic because you know the behavior is bad. In the real world, you cannot do something about that, but you can recognize the behavior in K-Dramas."

How well K-Dramas are able to provide us a cathartic cry, and I believe many of us, if not all of us, have experienced that while watching them. The key word is cathartic, which is what the clinician is trying to get across to her client in *Be Melodramatic* when the client questions what is wrong with her, trying to find a reason behind her emotions. I explain to people that our emotions are there, what we are feeling is what we are feeling, and it's okay not to be okay. When we question our emotions, it goes against the grain of what comes naturally. Preventing or avoiding something that is natural can make it so much more difficult. Here's an example. Have you ever been really hungry but had to delay eating for whatever circumstances, so that by the time it came for you to eat, you didn't feel hungry anymore? You waited so long to eat that your body got used to it and you felt numb. It's only when you finally get to eating that your body caves in and alerts you once again you were starving and needed the food.

The same goes for emotions. Perhaps you've walked around feeling very emotional, like you were holding back tears, but then suppressed them long enough that you ended up feeling numb and forgot what you were feeling in the first place. Once you avoid your emotions long enough, you forget you have them, and thus also become numb to the happy emotions that human beings need to experience. So if you suppress emotions thinking that it's the stronger thing to do or it's best not to show "weakness" being emotional—as it happens in Asian culture—you're missing out on feeling joy in your life. Healthy emotionality does not mean always being cheerful or showing positive emotions constantly. There's no such thing as being happy all the time, every minute of the day. When someone tells me they're always happy, I question it, though you can certainly feel content on a daily basis. But when I refer to healthy emotionality, it means expressing all the types of feelings you may be experiencing, even the unpleasant ones. The full range of emotions, from negative to positive, is normal.

I really mean it when I tell folks much of my work entails an "emotions 101" class where I help clients sort through what they're feeling by first naming and accepting them. Research indicates that crying releases oxytocin (the love, bonding hormone) and endorphins (one of the happy hormones). These feel-good chemicals alleviate and ease our pain and anguish. Crying also helps us feel calm, which boosts our physical well-being. It's important to understand that crying isn't only for times when you're sad, grieving, or empathizing with someone else's pain or sorrow. In fact, there are many more times we cry because we're happy, feeling loved or touched by someone or something. We can also cry because we're stressed, anxious, or frustrated.

Of course, what helps us understand the effectiveness of healthy emotionality are the mental health condition's themes throughout K-Dramas that I can pull out in my deep dives to educate clients and followers. K-Dramas do a beautiful job helping us see things outside of ourselves, where we don't feel as alone because someone else is experiencing the conflict or stressor and we can learn from it. There's a saying from me that I shared on social media that went viral: "If you can't stop watching K-Dramas, it's because they're healing your grief and trauma. A dose of a K-Drama a day shows you coping mechanisms that help you feel okay." K-Dramas are in no way a means to replacing therapy, though folks will sometimes say otherwise. However, they can provide examples of healthy coping and life skills, even helping you process emotions and situations that you otherwise wouldn't have seen on your own in real life.

When I was growing up, I felt like I was always walking on eggshells because of my strict upbringing. I recall holding back so much stress and anxiety, trying to be perfect but not having the outlet to express my emotions at home because of Korean cultural norms. There were times I did try to share with my parents, how I was struggling emotionally with my bicultural identity or the pressure they put on me regarding school and my extracurriculars. However, I was immediately shushed, shamed, or disciplined for what my parents (and elders) saw as complaining or being ungrateful. It was stifling, but that was the Korean way, so I held things in. This is not normal. We are human beings who are born to communicate in every way, both verbally and nonverbally. When I started watching K-Dramas, they gave me the safe space to feel and express all those emotions from childhood that I kept buried away. It was so cathartic and still is. I really felt detached from myself before watching K-Dramas, and in my research I have heard this from others as well. They didn't know what belongingness felt like until they started watching K-Dramas.

I'm referring to the belongingness in our emotions, owning them for what they are, with all the difficulty and the complexity they bring to our lives. After all, the more familiar we are with our emotions, the more we feel comfortable sitting with them to figure out how to navigate our lives with them. It helps us realize that they're nothing to be afraid of. Whether we know it or not, we are constantly thinking about our mental health, how we are feeling, how people make us feel. Psychological well-being is about how stressors and life events impact our brains, such as trauma and joyous occasions. Mental health is about how well we are balancing or not balancing life stressors with our own resilience. There's nothing linear about it; if you can picture mental health, it is a circle (think circle of life).

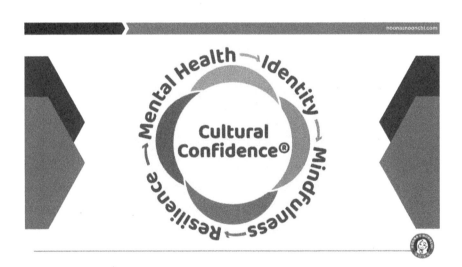

That's mental health in a nutshell. Mental health is health. As the World Health Organization (WHO) says, there is no health without mental health.

When folks ask me how K-Dramas relate to mental health, I tell them K-Dramas reflect real life in a dramatic way. After all it is a drama. The scenarios aren't realistic per se, but at the core, the themes, messages, and character emotions and reactions are indeed. I also get asked which K-Dramas are directly related to mental health. To be facetious, I ask how much time they have, because I could list every K-Drama out there. Yes, I do like to be funny because I want you to know how normal it is to talk about your mental health. Much of my work is to normalize it and break through the stigma for any change to happen, both in your life and systemically. I have so many stories to share of how people are in awe, baffled even as to how moved they are when watching K-Dramas.

Here's a story about what those emotional expressions can look like in one's life. A transracial adoptee named Rick who's Korean and Black told me he decided to start watching K-Dramas in the pandemic because he wanted to learn more about his Korean culture. He found out by mistake that he was adopted and didn't know he was Asian until age 16. He has quite a story, growing up thinking he was born of a white mother and Black father. Then one night he stumbled upon a family secret and realized his birth mother is Korean. It sounds like his own K-Drama. Because Rick had no exposure to his Korean culture growing up, he's been eager to find out all he can about a heritage he never knew he had. He started with 2020's *Itaewon Class* and then watched *Vagabond*. Both are more action oriented, which is the genre he thought enjoyed, until he saw 2021's *Hometown Cha-Cha-Cha*. Rick says this one is his favorite to date. It revealed emotions he didn't know he had, bringing him to tears, and they've been flowing ever since. Since seeing it, he's gotten more emotional and questions why. Even Rick's own wife of 10 years said she's never seen him this emotional and had questioned before this whether he was capable of emotions. Rick says this with a chuckle but realizes it's through K-Dramas that he's felt more connected to his emotions. Hence, the belongingness I was talking about.

In one of my corporate talks on K-Dramas for mental health, I happened to show a clip from *Hometown Cha-Cha-Cha* and hardly anyone in that conference had seen it. I set up the clip as best as I could; it showed the male lead breaking down after the female lead (his girlfriend) told him it's okay to feel the pain he's been experiencing and to let it out because she is there for him. It's a wonderful scene and I use it to show how we all crave validation, especially in our darkest moments. We don't necessarily need solutions. What we really want is to be heard, seen, and validated. That's the trade secret of therapy. I don't mind telling everyone this because that's the core of the human experience.

An executive from a mega corporation in my audience spoke up after I asked people to share any reflections after showing the *Hometown Cha-Cha-Cha* scene. She tentatively raised her hand, which I tend to expect in a corporate environment like this. What she shared touched everyone in the audience because of her frankness about the emotions she was experiencing. I recall her telling everyone, "I don't know what this is about, but I let one tear drop as I watched this scene. Just one tear, but I'm like, why? I don't know anything about this drama, let alone K-Dramas." Everyone in the audience chuckled softly, but she was honestly baffled by the one tear, indicating it wasn't like her to get even this emotional. Her colleagues, who know her, agreed, saying they were impressed with the one tear she showed and that she was honest about it. Comments like these are what I am used to because where there's a will, there's a way. Meaning, I can find a scene that gets you emotional or pulls at your heartstrings and makes a mark on you. It's because I believe in the power of K-Dramas storytelling and messaging. Otherwise, why would I be using it for mental health?

Because I personally believe in the power of K-Dramas, I feel that is why they are credible in my clinical work. When I speak to you about them, I am a human being above all else, so you're getting a very passionate, personal message from my heart. Period. I started using K-Dramas in my work because they moved me and made me a better person. I started using them as a tool, first to talk about mental health and break stigma, but second, to help people on a personal basis because the stories from K-Dramas reflect real life. What I was able to do personally that helped me explain the draw of K-Dramas to others was explain a clinical connection to the mental health conditions we are experiencing. I think that's what makes me believable. I am a trained mental health professional and I do lean on that to ensure I prove my point.

People have asked if other mediums could provide the same impact as K-Dramas, such as Chinese Dramas, Japanese Dramas, or other films and books. The short answer is yes, of course they can. We see it all the time. Other mediums make a tremendous impact on people and society. However, I'm coming from an angle that started out personal and then grew professional based on my Korean cultural heritage. It's quite a unique phenomenon to realize that Korean content can have such global appeal that it has benefited a country's economy, and that global leaders like the United States are taking notice.

3 | K-Dramas and Processing Grief

Grief is a complex cycle. There's no one way of experiencing or processing it. As a therapist, I find that grief is one of the most difficult things to help clients to navigate. We all have experienced it in one form or another. Grief isn't just a loss of a loved one, but a feeling, a loss of anything, from a job to physical safety to a relationship, and so much more. The Covid-19 pandemic was all about grief, the loss of normalcy as we knew it. When we went into a global lockdown, we felt such grief from the loss of a world as we had previously known it, where masks weren't required and we didn't have an unknown contagion among us. It's because of this grief that many sought solace at home through streaming sites that were readily accessible. It is there they found comfort from their pandemic grief in K-Dramas. In fact, I have encountered numerous K-Drama fans and followers who discovered K-Dramas just in the last couple of years. Because the world was grieving as the pandemic went into full swing in 2020, K-Dramas were a welcome distraction, with their heartwarming messages and family-friendly themes.

As with most things when it comes to mental health, grief is a complex cycle, not a linear progression. In K-Dramas, we get to see the grief cycle play out in various forms and not necessarily in any particular order. In my clinical experience, I have found that everyone grieves differently, and people can go through the grief cycle without rhyme or reason. According to the famous model by Swiss American psychiatrist Elisabeth Kubler-Ross, there are five stages in the grief cycle. Throughout the years, her approach has been extended to seven stages (as shown in the graphic here), which I found to be accurate in my work.

MODIFIED KUBLER-ROSS MODEL

THE 7 STAGES OF GRIEF

— **SHOCK** [initial paralysis at hearing the bad news]
— **DENIAL** [trying to avoid the inevitable]
— **ANGER** [frustrated outpouring of bottled-up emotion]
— **BARGAINING** [seeking in vain for a way out]
— **DEPRESSION** [final realization of the inevitable]
— **ACCEPTANCE & HOPE** [finally finding the way forward]
— **PROCESSING GRIEF** [navigating a changed POV]

CLAIMING GRIEF

K-Drama storytelling does a good job of outlining grief through characters' experiences to provide examples for people on how to navigate their own grief in real life. On one of my Instagram reels that went viral (nearly three million views), many people indicated that K-Dramas helped them through their grief—mainly due to the loss of loved ones—and many even cited specific series. Through watching a variety of situations in K-Dramas where characters encountered grief, viewers gave themselves permission and space to claim their grief, which in my clinical experience is a necessary first step to understand how to navigate through it.

Many people also share that they do not realize they are grieving until they watch K-Dramas and see a character going through the process. There's a process in narrative therapy called externalization, by which people separate themselves from the problem. For example, if someone has anxiety, through externalization they can look at their anxiety from a distance, apart from themselves. Then they can tackle the problem of anxiety, rather than feeling like they need to tackle themselves. In externalization, the person is never the problem; the problem is the problem. This is based on the narrative therapy model in family therapy created by Australian social worker Michael White and New Zealand social worker David Epston.

"K-Dramas helped me through my delayed grief process. I lost both my parents within a space of five weeks. I watched Good Doctor and the Hospital Playlist series, and I cried so much. Finally had to deal with the loss. Watching and seeing the characters grieving made me feel like it's okay to not be okay."

—*Noona's Noonchi follower*

Move to Heaven, 2021

When we watch K-Dramas, it's easier to externalize "the problem" from ourselves since we're watching someone else's story. Being able to do this helps us tackle our issues (in this case grief) in an effective way because we don't get all consumed in our problem. For instance, those who are grieving can tend to question why they're still struggling with grief after a long time, because grief has no specific end. When they see a grief storyline in a K-Drama, they're able to be more objective, an aspect of externalization because the grief they're seeing isn't about them. When it's not about us, it's easier for us to analyze and assess what's happening and perhaps come to a more beneficial, cohesive conclusion.

When it comes to understanding externalization surrounding the cycles of grief, 2021's *Move to Heaven* is a good example. The K-Drama was unique in that the main characters were trauma cleaners, and each episode had a different story surrounding characters who had already passed away. As you can gather from their job title, the trauma cleaners were responsible for cleaning up after a character's death, whether it was a murder or someone dying in their sleep. The main message of every episode was how each person's life is precious and everyone processes grief in their own personal way. With its different stories, *Move to Heaven* presented a variety of examples on how to grieve, and sent a poignant message that even death doesn't mean the end of your loved one's impact in your life. Their legacy can live on through your grief and your memories, which is perhaps the hope in such a heartbreaking season of life.

The various stories in this K-Drama let us get invested in the characters after their death because the trauma cleaners uncovered their stories, making externalization an easier process. What also made this K-Drama special was how the trauma cleaners uncovered "unfinished business" left by the deceased, and they followed through on what the deceased person had left behind and had not been able to finish prior to their death. This allowed their loved ones some reprieve from their grief, and perhaps a resolution that helped aid the grieving process. This was why I believe *Move to Heaven* left such a mark in viewers' lives and why it's one of my top K-Drama recommendations for grief. Grief is filled with many regrets—the could haves, would haves, or should haves. In a sense, the trauma cleaners in *Move to Heaven* were able to help clean up the regrets, which can take away some of the aches and pains of grief.

I want to share this poignant story that someone shared on my social media:

> "My husband passed away from Covid in March 2020. I was advised by a friend and cousin to try watching K-Dramas to keep my mind off my grief and depression. In December 2020, I tried to watch Crash Landing on You, and this started my love affair with K-Dramas. I am on my 180th series. The K-Dramas Chocolate and Hi Bye Mama are two of the best series on loss and grief."

Someone else responded to this person's message by saying she also lost her husband to Covid-19 in 2021 and started K-Dramas out of "curiosity." She indicated how it surprised her that they helped her so much and in unexpected ways. On the same thread, someone else shared that the K-Drama *Thirty-Nine* gave her reason to cry because she doesn't allow herself to cry much. She explained that she lost her father a couple of years earlier and pet losses followed that, as well as deaths in the extended family, so she was continuing to navigate her grief with the help of K-Dramas.

There's poignant belongingness in shared experiences. As folks were expressing on my social media, others were chiming in with their stories of grief and loss, and empathy and compassion ensued. Many brought me to tears because they found solace not only in these K-Drama stories of grief, but also in the fact that others understood what they were feeling. Grief can be very lonely because it's uncomfortable for those around you to know how to console or comfort. I tell people they can learn how to do that by watching these K-Dramas because you get to see not only how people are coping with grief, but also what the characters around them are doing to help those grieving.

Thirty-Nine, 2022

In *Thirty-Nine,* three best friends on the brink of turning 40 are experiencing life's joys and challenges together, including a terminal cancer diagnosis for one of them. This K-Drama showcased a beautiful example of womance (women friendships), and did a great job of depicting the poignancy of having loved ones rally behind someone with only months to live and power their way through their own grief that began the minute they learned of the cancer diagnosis.

Cancer is one of those very sad things we hear about it and is more common than we want. Doctors have told me it's one of the hardest things for medical providers to deal with. So viewing a K-Drama that focuses on how people deal with a loved one's cancer diagnosis is an important way to gain greater understanding in the grief surrounding it. We get to experience the cycle of grief with these women, as hard as it can be. Many other wonderful K-Dramas deal with grief, but I have found *Thirty-Nine* to be the one that stands out most when it comes to understanding and processing grief. It demonstrates how each character grieves differently, in their own unique way, because each person is unique. More importantly, it shows that grief can even contain moments of joy and excitement, and that one can learn to accept their terrible circumstances in a way that works for them to live their life the way they choose. Here are the dialectics again, where opposite emotions can manifest.

I have seen many people dictate what another person's grief should look like. When people are hurting, family members may think someone isn't grieving enough or showing enough emotion or care in the way they believe they should. *Thirty-Nine* provided a good scenario to use in similar cases in real life, including the perspective of the patient, who likely held the brunt of the grief in knowing she would be dying in just months, and grieving for her loved ones ahead of time because she knew how sad they would be. Jung Chan Young's experience as the cancer patient character was shown in conjunction with the reactions of those around her.

I use *Thirty-Nine* as my go-to for grief these days because it effectively presents the way its characters are experiencing all the various stages of grief. *Thirty-Nine* also showed how loved ones honored Chan Young's wish not to pursue further treatment than was necessary so she could live her final days with the quality of life as she wanted. That is not easy. As we can imagine in real life, this decision can be met with quite a lot of resistance. I've experienced it in my extended family when my uncle wanted his wife, my aunt, to continue treatment, but she wanted to stop when her end was near. The family was in disarray over what my aunt wanted for herself, versus what they wanted, which was to keep her alive as long as they possibly could. I have seen this tear families apart. The precious little time left can be filled with strife as family members' own grief trumps anything else. It certainly is understandable, but becomes one of the biggest regrets a family can have once their loved one has passed. *Thirty-Nine's* example was how I feel as a clinician. Things should be done to honor the patient's wishes. Her best friends even organized a party for her to see everyone she wanted to see, thus in a sense fulfilling Chan Young's wish to be at her own funeral.

Be Melodramatic, 2017

Also known as *Melo Is My Nature*, this K-Drama offers a beautifully poignant depiction of grief, also within a support system of female best friends. One of the main characters, Eun Jung, lost her fiancé to cancer, and in the depths of her despair she attempts suicide. After her suicide attempt and hospitalization, her best friends decide to move in with her and her brother, to ensure Eun Jeong's safety and take care of her, without telling her this directly. We as the viewers are to conclude this is due to her even-keeled, stoic personality. They want to give her space but continue worrying when they see Eun Jung speaking to no one on many occasions. The viewers know Eun Jung is speaking to her fiancé, whom she "sees" and "speaks" with as if he is there.

Following her suicide attempt, Eun Jung shows various stages of grief. Prior to that, it's a good assumption that she hadn't been coping well, suppressing everything and holding it in due to her natural temperament. In a moment of hopelessness, loneliness, and isolation, as she despairs in silence, she attempts to take her life. I am reiterating this part of the story—which happens early on—because it's important for us to note how unresolved or unprocessed grief can bring us to a point where the darkness is overwhelming and can shade our judgment or rationale completely.

As she returns to her regular schedule, and copes by speaking with her fiancé's ghost, we see her experience denial, bargaining, and teetering back and forth in silent anger. The crucial moment comes at the end of episode nine, when she sees video footage of herself speaking to her fiancé's ghost (no one is visible with her) and realizes that she's depressed. This realization leads her back to reality, where she courageously comes before her best friends and her brother and asks them for help, saying she's having a tough time. I point out this scene repeatedly as an excellent example of the healing process. Your support system in times of adversity is critical. But equally critical is asking for help despite the depth of pain, hurt, and sorrow you are experiencing. Expressing your grief in the hardest of moments is a huge part of your healing journey.

Suppressing tears can lead to sickness, and this is what happens to Eun Jung early in her grief when she is perhaps still in shock, leading to her suicide attempt. Although we want to be strong, especially in Asian culture where expressing emotion isn't endorsed, it is not healthy or normal to do so. I want this to be a reminder that, in any stage of the grief cycle we are in, we can feel so numb that self-harm seems to be the only way to experience pain, which is not an effective way of coping. Although Eun Jung finally reveals her feelings before her support system, she still has a hard journey ahead of her, as we see when she seeks therapy. Thus we see Eun Jung continue to struggle, but now it is openly with tears of anger, sorrow, confusion, and guilt. Many emotions come out in therapy, and therapy is by no means easy, but is a way to help someone navigate their healing and process with a person who can guide them through it.

I have heard many stories from clients and followers where in their grief, they are blinded by such powerful sadness they don't take care of themselves, or self-harm unwittingly, as shown by example in *Be Melodramatic*. A former client told me about a friend who experienced such intense grief, she ended up in the hospital for dehydration and an overdose of sleeping pills. The patient had her engagement broken just a few weeks before the wedding. She was devastated, to say the least, and didn't eat or drink for days despite coaxing and pleas from her family. She ended up fainting one morning and had to be taken to the hospital, where she remained for almost a week and was even put on suicide watch due to her vulnerable state. I believe this was not so much a clear-cut case of self-harm but rather self-neglect, due to the intense grief she felt over her loss. Her fiancé wasn't dead, but she lost a relationship, an engagement, and what she perceived to be her future marriage. The intense pain, sadness, and sorrow we may experience from grief can cause us to behave in ways we never imagined. It's important to remember that everyone handles their grief differently and we cannot tell others how to grieve.

As I mentioned previously, dialectics are an important aspect of understanding our emotional well-being, particularly grief, where people can be in despair. Dialectics refer to opposite experiences and emotions that can be felt at the same time. Dialectical behavioral therapy is one of the modalities I use often in my work. Through the emotional struggles of K-Drama characters, people can see that grief can coexist with other emotions. One of my followers shared that the biggest lesson for her from K-Dramas pertaining to grief was that her "joy and sadness can coexist." As she explained, "It sounds like a contradiction, but K-Drama tears can be healing and that has helped me process my grief." My response was that the contradiction she speaks of is normal and an example of dialectics at play. It may be a clinical modality, but dialectics are part of everyday life and a way of confirming that we are normal because we cannot compartmentalize our emotions, even though we would like to at times. What's normal is undergoing many of them at the same time, as contradictory as that might feel.

Finally, what lies in grief is hope. Hope is something I'll discuss in more detail later when I talk about mindfulness and resilience. That is exactly why I tell clients to work through their grief. It doesn't have to be all or nothing or either-or. It's not all black and white—there can be shades of gray in mental health. Feeling it all, from heartbreak to hopefulness, is mental health. Going through grief can feel unbearable, but the hope is that you navigate through it minute by minute, day by day, going through the grief cycle toward the goal of finding hope in your sorrow. Hope is what sustains us through our rock-bottom moments, so we must have that and bring it out when we can. I hear a lot from clients who have experienced such terrible loss in their lives that they are a different person post-grief. They were someone else pre-grief, and now their grief is part of their identity. I find this makes sense, and K-Drama character development shows it beautifully. It is actually why we keep watching. We want to see the character deal effectively with their grief, hoping they will feel better. We have hope for our beloved K-Drama characters to be happy. That hope for their happiness gives us an understanding of what hope feels like. Because it feels good, we have that yearning for it in our own lives.

Top K-Dramas for navigating grief:
- *Move to Heaven*
- *Goblin*
- *Chocolate*
- *Hi Bye, Mama*
- *Thirty-Nine*
- *Go Back Couple*
- *If You Wish Upon Me*
- *Call It Love*
- *Thirty, But Seventeen*
- *Be Melodramatic*
- *Divorce Attorney Shin*
- *Uncontrollably Fond*

4

K-Dramas and Korean *Han*

When talking about grief in the context of K-Dramas, it's important to understand the Korean version of grief and sorrow which is referred to as *Han*. In fact, I believe Han is the foundation of the emotional experience we see in the stories and characters. Han is another uniquely Korean concept that presents more difficult emotions felt at one's core: deep-rooted resentment, regret, sorrow, even bitterness. Han is what Koreans feel inside (whether they know it or not), especially the older population because they've lived through the tougher times in Korea, from the Korean war to a contentious government to economic turmoil. Han is also about grief, particularly collective grief, and loss of identity especially in this older population. I believe Han is passed down from generation to generation, like intergenerational trauma.

Han can also be controversial, because some people believe it is not part of Korean society but is a modern concept that came out of the Japanese occupation of Korea. In fact, experts and researchers indicate that Han holds different meanings in the Korean diaspora. Interestingly, South Koreans do not find significance in Han, seeing it instead as a part of history. On the other hand, Korean Americans find a great deal of meaning in Han, emphasizing its importance in cultural and collective identity. From my point of view, this certainly all feels valid and I won't discount the vast diversity of perspectives in the Korean diaspora. But I will still point out that Han is a common thread in K-Drama storytelling. It seems to be the anchor of the story. K-Dramas showcase Han through the back stories of the characters—detailing their past hurts, traumas, sorrows, joys, and successes—while at the same time showing how they got to where they are now, or what prompted their fall from grace.

From this viewpoint, I am led to conclude that Han very much exists in Korean society. It makes sense because Korea has a sad, oppressed history and was the target of the powerful nations of Japan and China seeking control. Han can also include a sense of injustice and feeling wronged, and can motivate someone to change their circumstances and fight for their rights. The revenge theme in K-Dramas has been quite popular as of late, and it resonates with folks because they want to see justice served and the corrupt punished. The audience feels compassion for the underdog and likes to see characters with whom they empathize come out on top.

The Han emotions of sadness, sorrow, grief, and resentment may sound negative, but it depends on how you look at them. They are part of life, part of the human experience. From a mental health perspective, they are the balance of the more upbeat emotions that can build our resilience. We need that balance. We cannot be erring on the side of the positive all the time, or vice versa.

I am not a historian, nor equipped to fully explain Korea's history as an expert. However, what I know about Han both as a Korean and as a mental health professional is that it stems from Korea's turbulent and sad history as I mentioned earlier. It's in the essence of Korea and is threaded throughout Korean society, history, and geography. In fact, there are some who believe that Han is in the blood of all Koreans.

Those of you who watch K-Dramas most likely understand what Han looks like because you see it displayed in the characters. Now you have a term for it. I believe Han is very critical to understanding the core messaging in K-Dramas. Through its embodiment of difficulty, Han has provided a pathway to building resilience. Han resonates with hope. Because of it, Korean society has worked hard to overcome its vulnerabilities to become a nation that's put itself on the map. It would therefore be expected that the Korean writers of K-Dramas would write Han into their stories to reflect the way characters are overcoming their demons, trials, and tribulations, to have a stronger sense of self and to make their own mark in their society in K-Drama land.

Han is also an example of a dialectic in a less obvious way. The tough emotions surrounding Han have ended up fueling Korean society to power through those tough times and prove themselves. Han is not only about regret but redemption as well. During the Korean war,

Koreans lost their families in their escape from North Korea to the south, but the redemption is perhaps how they have lived out their lives in working hard and creating a new life of freedom for themselves for the sake of their families who didn't make it to freedom with them. It's why I tell folks that making decisions based on regret is a terrible way to live. There's got to be reciprocity—give and take, push and pull—to allow for redemption to reveal itself in order for a healthy way of life. Again, mental health isn't linear; there's a circular causality to it.

Han is so complex that even Koreans have trouble explaining it, but they feel it. That's how it can be, at times, to explain the mental health benefits of K-Dramas. It is significant that K-Dramas depict both regret and redemption, dialectics that are polar opposites that can exist together. The characters in K-Dramas are a wonderful example of everyone's complexity; people are both good and bad at times, and we don't have to be defined by the worst event or trauma in our life or by wrongdoing. We can aspire to be much more than that.

Start-Up, 2020

I'll share an example of what Han looks like through the lens of K-Dramas by using 2020's *Start-Up* as an example. That this Netflix K-Drama was a hit is particularly due to the popularity of the second male lead, Han Ji Pyeong. There sure was Han in Han Ji Pyeong (pun intended). This self-made millionaire venture capitalist built himself from the ground up. He came from nothing: an orphan taken care of by the grandmother of the female lead character, Seo Dalmi, with whom he became pen pals when she was a teenager. He showed Han in his orphan upbringing, having aged out of the foster care system and having to live on his own. What he had going for him was his brains. With his gift for understanding how to invest money, he found success as an adult by becoming a rich VC, and thus had the wherewithal to invest money in others' start-ups. Though he comes across as an obnoxious know-it-all, he nevertheless has a heart of gold. Those opposing characteristics can go hand in hand—that's the Han in Han Ji Pyeong. He resented his upbringing, grieved perhaps a happier childhood where he could feel loved and be loved by parents. Yet he directed that Han into his success and was later able to help many start-ups turn into successful companies. The maternal figure in his life knew it all boiled down to his being lonely, and she loved him the best way she could so he could work through his Han loneliness and find happiness in his life. That's not to say Han Ji Pyeong was unhappy; he was not, but he wasn't happy either. That's what Han can look like. We see more than three dimensions; our emotional well-being can look more like four dimensions. The prism of Han can look bright and shiny or dark and dull, depending on how the light hits it.

Our Blues, 2022

What a beautiful K-Drama this is—very layered, with an ensemble cast and incorporating different but intersecting storylines that are somehow all connected by someone or something. For the sake of helping you understand Han a little more, the character I want to focus on is Lee Dong Seok, played by Lee Byung Hun. From the moment we see him he is angry and frustrated much of the time. He speaks harshly to those around him, except the woman he is in love with. He directs the majority of his anger at his estranged mother, with whom he lives in the same vicinity but doesn't speak with. We are led to assume he's hurt from something that happened in the past during his childhood, but his mother's silence is deafening. Their relationship is what I've been using lately in my workshops when addressing intergenerational trauma (explored in the next chapter).

At the core of intergenerational trauma is Han. In the story, Dong Seok's mother knows her son is angry at her but continues along her way regardless. Dong Seok's anger is well known in the community since he's obvious in the way he addresses her. The Han in Dong Seok stems from what he feels is the unjust way he was not protected by his mother after she married his stepfather and how he was bullied by his stepbrothers. Dong Seok shows his bitterness toward his mother because he feels she chose his stepfather and stepbrothers over him. It explains why we see him causing trouble as a teen growing up, being troubled himself, and perhaps feeling neglected by his own mother and desiring her attention as much as possible. Dong Seok's Han stems from what I described above: that Han is a deep-seated sadness, sorrow, regret, and anger because of something he believed he deserved but didn't get to have. Han includes the feeling of being unjustly treated and wanting to take back what one believes is theirs. Also, since Han is at the root of Korean identity, it has an intergenerational impact, being passed down to subsequent generations, and Dong Seok's Han stems from his mother.

Again, Han is a core, underlying message of K-Dramas. It's why many people resonated with *Our Blues* when it came to Dong Seok's relationship with his mother. Clients, followers, and other people have indicated how much they resonated with the moment (spoiler) Dong Seok shares his thoughts at his mother's deathbed. In a sense, he was releasing his Han in that moment of her death when he lets his tears flow after holding them for decades. He admits that all he wanted was to be her son, and to hold her like he's doing as she dies of cancer. Several followers messaged me that they broke down watching that scene because their parent died before they could express their love and forgiveness. However, their own Han held the bitterness to the end, building a wall of stoicism to prevent further hurt from their childhood.

There's a poignant moment in episode 20 where Dong Seok admits his sorrow and shares how he feels with his mother, telling her she took his own mother away years ago, the mother he wanted to be with and always wanted to have. He asks her how she could be like that to him, her own son. I like to point out to families—particularly the second generation, who struggle understanding their parents—is her emotionally raw response to him. I believe it's rare to get such a response and most likely many of us from immigrant families will never hear from our own parents and families what she shared in this episode. She tells her son, in her own words, what immigrant parents experience but cannot share because they weren't provided the language or support to navigate their own grief and trauma. Dong Seok's mother says she wasn't in her right mind following the death of her own husband (his father) and daughter (his sister). The mother indicates it was her fault his sister died, and she wanted to keep surviving so she married his stepfather and thought it was enough to give her son a roof over his head and food to eat.

This is at the core of the immigrant mentality. Survive, not thrive, and just provide the basic necessities for their offspring to live. But the second generation wants their parents' emotional and social presence and attention, which is why there exists such a cultural conflict. Dong Seok responds with tears but doesn't say anything as she tells him she wasn't fit to be his mother, so she did the unforgiveable and stepped back. This, my friends, is what we tend to see our elders do. They carry such guilt and shame that they do not know how to express their Han, so it is shoved deeper and deeper within. In their quest to protect their offspring, they carry that burden all around, which translates into a distance that the younger generation struggle with.

Our Blues is a recent drama, so it has been useful for me to repeatedly discuss Dong Seok's relationship with his mother and the moments in episode 20 because I believe they're significant to understanding the intergenerational dynamic between immigrant parents and their children, how Han can manifest, and how to learn from this storytelling example to better understand our parents and families. This is the beauty of a K-Drama or any medium where we get to see multiple perspectives of a storyline that we otherwise do not get to see in real life. Parents or grandparents or other elders may never share their feelings or thoughts with you, and therefore there may not be a resolution to your Han. However, the hope is (there's always hope) that we, ourselves, can shift that Han into something that is more about thriving, not just surviving. I continue to see this pattern today where the aging population holds on to their Han, which prevents them from making connections with the younger generation and is therefore misinterpreted by the younger folks who are hurt by what they see as lack of affection when it really is the opposite.

I believe that Han was what sustained Korean society to get to where it is today. I share about it because this subtle yet quite profound emotional sentiment resonates in every K-Drama. We see the Han in characters striving to thrive and then when they get there in true K-Drama fashion, we see Han turn into hope. Although some would say that Han is such deep-rooted sorrow and regret at the core of the Korean people, I don't believe that Han is the main emotional experience for people. Otherwise, how can we explain the success Korea has seen today with its content, beauty, and food? The Han is something Korean society navigates while hoping for a better tomorrow—hoping that their hard work comes to fruition, toiling through a history of turmoil and turbulence so that hope will balance out the Han. The hope reflects Korea today in the eyes of the rest of the world. To dispel the bitterness and sadness of life, Koreans toiled on their soil to find a way to rid themselves of the Han, seeking the pursuit of happiness, as we may call it. They found themselves building and promoting Korean culture such as K-Pop and K-Dramas in a way that was effective and empowering.

5

K-Dramas and Healing Our Traumas

The healing journey is very much a part of the K-Drama experience, so I want to tackle the topic of trauma sooner rather than later. Trauma is defined as any frightening, distressful event or experience in one's life. What may be traumatic to you may not be traumatic to me. This is important to understand. In real life, healing from trauma can be a lifelong journey. Coming from a trauma-informed lens, I hold the perspective that trauma is a part of everyone's life. All of us have experienced trauma in one form or another. I am used to the looks I get when I start discussing trauma in workshops (not so much in therapy, for obvious reasons). People avert their gaze when I talk about trauma because it is uncomfortable. It can also be triggering, especially when I tie it into specific examples via K-Drama clips. However, as my noonchi will guide me, I can pivot a conversation when I need to, depending on reactions, or delve deeper based on people's reactions. Numerous times I have had to dig very deep to figure out someone's trauma because they themselves weren't able to share it or know they had experienced something that turned out to be traumatic that they were suppressing. This is where K-Dramas come in.

Because trauma is not easy even for a therapist to speak about, especially in a setting as a corporate speaker, showing K-Drama clips can break the ice. Pre-pandemic, I would talk about how K-Dramas show raw examples of trauma, but folks didn't really buy into it so my explanation of trauma and examples thereof would be somewhat dry. However, with the boom of K-Dramas and their global appeal, I am able to speak more freely, especially accompanied with a K-Drama clip to get my point across. Because I'm discussing trauma, I am cognizant of what I am showing, so I work hard at featuring a clip that doesn't so much show the actual trauma incident but instead reveals how the character deals with it and heals from it. K-Dramas consistently show various types of traumas, and discussing them in my work has been useful in helping many people. My specialty is also in trauma as a Certified Clinical Trauma Professional because, from a trauma-informed perspective, I see it frequently in my work both within and outside of therapy. K-Dramas have become a tremendous benefit in my work in helping people deal with trauma.

Racial Trauma

In a post-pandemic world, the Asian American Native Hawaiian Pacific Islander (AANHPI) community in the United States has elevated their voice, particularly amid anti-Asian hate. It's important for me to talk about this in my book because racism is a big part of the mental health crisis. Being in the field of mental health, I find racism and the trauma surrounding to be a part of my daily life both personally and professionally. Racial trauma, also known as race-based traumatic stress, refers to the effects of racism on our mental and physical health. It's important to know that racial trauma can impact us even as children, which seems to have been a common experience for those of us who are middle-aged and older, since racism was rarely addressed back in our childhood days. Racial trauma can stem from numerous causes, including first-hand experience, vicariously, and indirectly from hearing about an incident on the news, on social media, from friends, other sources.

From a clinical perspective, the global pandemic was perhaps the first time the AANHPI community broached the topic of racism and racial trauma in general conversations. In my line of work, I would discuss it with experts and academics, but hearing it openly discussed is, I believe, a step closer to breaking the stigma surrounding mental health in our community. Racial trauma due to anti-Asian hate was one of the most common subjects I addressed in my talks, sessions, and workshops over the last four years. I've shared this before, but what really helped me unwind and decompress after a difficult day talking about trauma, addressing trauma, tackling trauma with clients was watching a K-Drama episode or two.

There are several ways K-Dramas can help us manage and navigate through racial trauma. I'll start first with AANHPIs. Because we're talking about Korean dramas, they're representative of Asian culture. Therefore, we get to see Asian representation, which is important in order to feel seen, heard, and validated. Racism isn't portrayed in Korean dramas, understandably so, because South Korea (for the most part) is a homogenous country. Though it's more diverse now with so many foreigners living in South Korea, my focus right now is discussing racism as a systemic issue, which doesn't have an impact in South Korea, so we don't see it in K-Dramas. Though episode 8 of 2019's *Itaewon Class* did show an example of racial discrimination toward the Black character Tony, K-Drama stories don't tend to depict racism. Why does this matter? Watching things that are positive and uplifting can help us escape, in a sense, from the racism in our real lives, albeit briefly. It provides respite from the real-life challenges that await us. K-Dramas are a far cry from the news, which can get depressing because "what bleeds, leads." I know this as a former journalist. K-Dramas, both directly and indirectly, can help us manage racial trauma because we see hope in a K-Drama (imaginary) world where racism doesn't exist. It's nice to live there for a while to give us some energy, and recharge our batteries.

Secondary Trauma

Secondary trauma is an indirect or secondhand experience of trauma. Secondary trauma can happen immediately after watching something traumatic on TV or in the media or hearing it described by a friend. People can also get secondary trauma from reading something online such as a social media post or an article. I spoke a lot about secondary trauma amid the pandemic, especially following the mass shootings throughout the United States and a tragedy like the Itaewon crowd crush in 2022. In light of pandemic times, with many people utilizing social media, secondary trauma was not an uncommon experience. After the tragic shootings, I took to my platform to speak and educate many on how secondary trauma is something we all need to look out for. It was timely because everything was unfolding in the news and on social media.

In 2022's *Twenty-Five Twenty-One,* secondary trauma is well displayed in episodes 15–16 in the character of journalist Baek Yi Jin, who covers the 9-11 terrorist attacks in New York City. I was glad to find a good example of secondary trauma so I could utilize it to get my point across. It's not necessarily that we can prevent secondary trauma, but we can most certainly be aware of how it manifests and how to manage it. As a reporter, Baek Yi Jin had the job to cover the continuing story surrounding 9-11 as it was unfolding. This included interviewing 9-11 survivors, first responders, rescue workers, crisis management officials, and whoever else was willing to speak and share their story. Not only did Baek Yi Jin hear disturbing accounts, especially from survivors and victims' families, but he also had to face their anger, grief, and trauma over what they experienced. Through it all, as part of his responsibility as a professional journalist, Baek Yi Jin had to remain calm because it's important for a journalist to be neutral and get the facts. This is especially challenging in a time of crisis and tragedy. Although Baek Yi Jin is aware of how many horrors he's hearing on a day-to-day basis, he keeps going for the sake of the job. This is why he began to show signs of post-traumatic stress and at one point displayed post-traumatic stress disorder (PTSD), which he hints at when he speaks to his girlfriend, Na Hee Do.

Here's another reason why K-Dramas can show us so much. We don't see Baek Yi Jin experience secondary trauma until toward the end of the K-Drama, after he covers 9-11. As viewers, we've gotten to know the character before the secondary trauma and then we observe him afterward. This makes it a straightforward case study for me to show in my sessions and workshops. In terms of everything happening in the world during the pandemic, secondary trauma is something I want everyone to understand because I am seeing it more often. Many K-Drama viewers assumed Baek Yi Jin was experiencing PTSD, but PTSD is a result of a direct trauma event in your life or witnessing a terrifying event, and Baek Yi Jin did not directly experience the actual 9-11 terrorist attack. He was being traumatized each time he heard a tragic story or graphic account from a 9-11 survivor. Although there was some criticism that the show handled 9-11 in a sensationalized way, I focused on what it could teach everyone about secondary trauma in a character they had grown to love in a K-Drama they enjoyed. The many Asian American journalists I worked with during this time of anti-Asian hate reminded me of Baek Yi Jin. They were covering stories after stories on racist incidents, attacks, and events and they were in need of trauma support. Working with these journalists has been such as privilege since I started my career as a broadcast journalist and understand how trauma exposure takes its toll. In fact, in the latter part of the pandemic, I educated many journalists on how I was also seeing vicarious trauma in their emotional symptoms.

Historically, vicarious trauma manifested in medical and clinical providers (like me) and first responders working with people in pain or feeling fearful, or survivors of traumatic events such as 9-11 or victims of anti-Asian hate. However, in recent months, many journalists, particularly Asian Americans, are showing signs of vicarious trauma as well, due to covering so many of these stories during a short period of time.

Intergenerational Trauma

Intergenerationality—the interactions between members of different generations—is core to our K-Dramas because this is a significant aspect of Asian culture. All K-Dramas show various aspects of intergenerationality, which means we see many examples of intergenerational trauma. I discuss this in my core workshops because it is part of our Asian identity and has been a mainstay in conversations across all communities, particularly AANHPIs. While we discussed intergenerational trauma more often than racial trauma pre-pandemic, it is because of what transpired from the pandemic that AANHPIs (and other ethnic communities) have had to address international trauma, also known as the "elephant in the room."

Intergenerational trauma is a term that was first coined by psychologists when they recognized it in the children of Holocaust survivors. Also known as transgenerational trauma, this is the trauma, both psychological and physiological, surrounding an event, experience, or incident experienced by one generation that gets passed down to subsequent generations. Examples of events that produce intergenerational trauma include global pandemics (i.e., Covid-19), natural disasters, and societal tragedies (i.e., school shootings). In terms of the Asian community, intergenerational trauma stems from such things as the Korean War, the Vietnam War, and acculturation, which is the process that results from immigrating from your country of origin to a host country. It involves social, psychological, and cultural adjustment to your host culture. An example is my parents' experience when they immigrated, with me as a baby, from South Korea to the United States in 1974. Acculturation is what I see in my work as the biggest contributor to intergenerational trauma because there's so much entailed in that process, from the micro to the macro level.

How does intergenerational trauma correlate with K-Dramas? Let me go back to its definition. Intergenerational trauma refers to the trauma experienced by one generation and how their behavior from the impact of their trauma affects the generations following them. This is what I would call a core theme in most K-Dramas because it's such an integral part of the Asian narrative. I'll provide a few K-Drama examples here to help you understand what it can look like and how I use K-Drama examples to help my clients.

The Good Bad Mother, 2023

This K-Drama was popular, but some folks couldn't watch it because the stark example of intergenerational trauma was too triggering.

I'll do a deep dive into this one. In the first episode, we see the main character, the mother, Jin Young Soon, experience a horrific tragedy. Her husband is murdered, but the perpetrators stage his death as a suicide; she suspects foul play, but the prosecutor hired to take on her case is corrupt, paid off the perpetrators so he knows the terrible truth. Young Soon loses her pig farm in the process. The most terrible aspect of all this is that she is pregnant with her first child. Research indicates that trauma can get passed down in the womb via the stress hormone cortisol, which can reach the baby via the placenta. This is how the K-Drama begins, so viewers see her trauma unfold, along with its aftermath. Hence the title *The Good Bad Mother*. Because of the atrocities she experienced, she does everything she can to ensure her son has a good life, so she is harsh to the point that many viewers struggled with her parenting methods. For example, she won't let her son finish his dinner for fear that he would fill his stomach too much, which could put him in a food coma and prevent him from working through the night on his studies. She also doesn't allow him to have any fun and pushes him to be a lawyer so he can live a good life. Young Soon's one-track mind is typical of what I see in Asian families from parents who, in their desperation, go to extremes to protect their children from experiencing what they did. It's also a way to prevent themselves from furthering their trauma because it's a parent's worst nightmare to be seeing your child suffer.

The Good Bad Mother presents a very good example of intergenerational trauma. In fact, it's the only K-Drama I can think of that portrays this trauma as its core theme. I've pointed out to clients and followers that we get to see how the trauma of one generation, the mother, begins and then proceeds to impact the next generation, her son, because every decision the mother makes is founded on her trauma experience. There is no thought of seeking professional help (i.e., therapy), so her means of survival is being a "good bad mother." There are the dialectics again: opposite elements coexisting at the same time. The reason intergenerational trauma is referred to as a cycle is that the pattern of behavior can continue repeating itself until a family member in one generation stops that pattern of behavior. What this K-Drama does well is realistically show the agony of the mother parenting her son harshly so he can live a good life. There are some difficult scenes, I'll admit, and people asked me things like, "How can a mother do this to her son?" Even for a therapist, it's tough to explain, especially for those who are not Asian, because this is an aspect of the culture we are used to. But as is so often the case in K-Dramas, we get a comprehensive look at the character. We get to see behind the scenes of the harsh parenting and are reminded where the mother is coming from. After perhaps a terribly mean comment from the mother (or a parent in other K-Dramas), we as viewers will then see the mother crying her eyes out because she knows how hurtful she's being to her child. That, my friends, is something we rarely get in real life and is why K-Dramas can be so helpful in our coping. We are able to see another perspective without realizing it.

Something in the Rain, 2018

Many other K-Dramas show intergenerational trauma in different ways. *Something in the Rain* centers on the relationship between Yoon Jinah (Son Yejin of *Crash Landing on You* fame) and Seo Joonhee (Jung Haein)—a relationship Jinah's parents highly disapprove of, particularly her mother. Even before the relationship is revealed (they hide it for a while), we see Jinah's mother rant and rave that Jinah is not married, and she's been setting up her daughter with men she herself approves of. Jinah's mother acts similarly to the mother in *Good Bad Mother,* with some atrocious behavior that may appall you and may look like abuse. That's the hard part in all this. The behavior that stems from intergenerational trauma isn't at all healthy and yes, the traumatized person's behavior can be abusive. Aside from the fact that Jinah is older, her mother thinks Joonhee is not good enough due to his family background.

Ironically, the family has been close to Jinah's family, and they grew up together. Folks often tend to reference this K-Drama when it comes to intergenerational trauma because they have a hard time accepting the mother's behavior, and I don't blame them. Many clients and followers have shared that it's very difficult to watch and that they were angered by the mother's behavior toward her daughter. We don't get to see much of a behind-the-scenes redemption in the mother as we normally do in the antagonist in a K-Drama, and it's hard to understand where the mother is coming from. The deep dive I provided on this is that the mother was still traumatized herself. She appears to be in a good marriage so it most likely stems not from her marriage but from her own mother's behavior toward her, and perhaps her own parents disapproved of her marriage.

A few followers have told me they wept so hard watching *Something in the Rain* realizing how much pain they were in due to their own mothers. Although they indicated it was hard to get through, they felt a safe space for an emotional release for the first time, and empathizing with Jinah helped begin their healing.

True Beauty, 2020

In this K-Drama, the mother of Lim Jookyung, the female protagonist, asks her daughter during a confrontation, "Do you want to end up doing what I'm doing?" Now that is a classic line from a traumatized parent in the cycle of intergenerational trauma. Jookyung and her mother were arguing about Jookyung enrolling in cosmetology school, and her mother prohibits her from following through. In another scene, the mother dumps all of Jookyung's precious makeup in the trash in one swift move. As viewers we find that horribly mean, but when you look closely at the mother's emotions, she is more sad than mad. Her daughter's passion for cosmetology is triggering. It seems ironic considering the mother is also a cosmetologist, but that's what intergenerational trauma looks like. A parent fears their child(ren) will end up like them or end up doing what they're doing, and they don't think they're good enough. This line of thinking stems from their own upbringing, particularly in the Asian culture, where even if you do accomplish something you are proud of, it's viewed simply as an expectation you are supposed to meet, and therefore not viewed as a success from a parent's point of view.

The Red Sleeve, 2021

This popular historical drama (loosely based on Korean history in the Joseon dynasty) provides an example of intergenerational trauma between a grandfather and grandson. The trauma of the grandfather, King Yeongjo, comes from the sensitivity surrounding his difficult upbringing by a concubine mother and how he came onto the throne. His actions throughout the drama stem from feeling insecure about his leadership, so he is constantly seeking to prove to everyone that he is truly the king and must be obeyed. He punishes anyone who questions his leadership, including his own grandson, who later becomes King Jeongjo. In some scenes he threatens to have his grandson—the heir to the throne—killed for what he believes is disobedience. The grandfather also refers to the conflicted feelings over the death of his son, whom he ordered to be executed for having a mental illness. The guilt he feels over this decision permeates his behavior, and his grandson is the one who must endure it.

Breaking the Trauma Cycle

Critical to tackling intergenerational trauma is learning how to break its cycle. That is the hope, and that is why I do what I do. However, it is not a one and done. Intergenerational trauma is complex, which also means its solutions are complex. Breaking the cycle is a daily part of how you adjust your behavior, monitor your thought patterns, and regulate your emotions so you are not falling into the same patterns as previous generations. The younger generation is at an advantage because there are more conversations now surrounding trauma and how to navigate it. The key is awareness, which brings about understanding. I look at patterns of behavior to understand how families can get off the hamster wheel of trauma where they keep spinning in unhealthy communication and attempts at coping. Explaining this in client sessions is one thing, but showing it through K-Drama scenes is an added benefit to get my point across.

The K-Drama examples I outlined above all show one very important aspect of intergenerational trauma: subsequent generations breaking the cycle. This is why K-Dramas are so powerful and positive. In the *Good Bad Mother,* the son seeks to avenge his father's murder and do what he can to bring the right folks to justice for the sake of finally living in peace with his mother. He directs the angst from his upbringing and perhaps his mother's harsh parenting to using his skills to create a new life and a better future for himself. The closeness he has with his mother comes after his accident (spoiler alert), where they are given a second chance to build a strong bond that changes the trajectory of both their lives.

Something in the Rain's female protagonist, though she struggled to find her footing and separate her values from that of her mother's, eventually discovers her own self-worth. She moves away from her family to Jeju Island, quits her job—a progressive move in Korean culture—and reunites with her boyfriend, Joon Hee. They had broken up due to the heated family conflict, but she pushes past that to define her life on her own terms.

In both *True Beauty* and *The Red Sleeve,* the female and male protagonist, respectively, follow through with their passion for their work. One element in breaking the cycle of trauma is confronting the conflict and working through it, addressing the elephant in the room. It also means standing firm in front of your parents or elders to show confidence and pride in your decisions and life choices. In *The Red Sleeve,* when the grandson becomes King Jeongjo he chooses to be the type of king he desires to be, particularly in being confident that he can lead. He didn't get to see this from his grandfather, but he sought his own leadership path because of what he grew up with.

Although I am pointing out these wonderful K-Drama examples of how the trauma cycle can indeed be broken, it is important for me to make sure you understand that we only see the happily-ever-after endings. Healing from trauma is an ongoing process, a lifelong journey. I am assuming that if the story in a particular K-Drama kept going, we would see the younger generation make mistakes and fall back into the pattern of behavior of their previous generation. What they have going for them is being keenly aware of what they want to change because they see that they do not want to repeat the behavior pattern of those before them.

6 | K-Dramas and Post-Traumatic Stress Disorder

Since we're talking about trauma, that means we must also address post-traumatic stress (PTS). To be clear, this is the stress reaction that happens following a traumatic event or incident, such as after a car accident, the death of a loved one, or a natural disaster such as a hurricane or, most recently, the historic global pandemic. Post-traumatic stress shows up in your fight-or-flight reaction, such as crying, or being very upset, physically sick, or nervous because of the trauma you experienced. All this is a normal reaction to something traumatic. It is not post-traumatic stress disorder (PTSD), a mental health disorder (mental illness)—at least not yet. PTS is common and generally goes away on its own with everyday stress-relieving and coping techniques.

Post-traumatic stress becomes PTSD when the symptoms do not go away and last over a month, and your usual destressing techniques do not work. Also, your daily functioning could be impaired because you're unable to think about anything else, are hypervigilant, and are having flashbacks of the traumatic event. It's important to note that, according to the PTSD Alliance, PTSD symptoms can begin immediately after the trauma or might show up weeks, months, or even years later. For example, I've diagnosed PTSD in the Asian community following the Atlanta spa shooting tragedy because this incident triggered reactions from a childhood trauma that individuals had experienced.

Several K-Dramas show fairly accurate portrayals of PTSD, which I have pointed out in my sessions and on social media. In fact, PTSD is one of the most talked about mental health disorders in recent months. I believe that has much to do with the state of everyone's mental health in the changed post-pandemic world. There's a growing understanding that PTSD does not apply only to war veterans, which was an assumption for so long. One of the first reels to go viral on Instagram was my reel on "K-Dramas that accurately portray PTSD." This chapter explores the K-Dramas that I believe are good examples of PTSD to help you understand what it looks like.

Rain or Shine, 2017

This K-Drama is loosely based on the 1995 Sampoong Department Store collapse that killed 502 people, the largest peacetime disaster in South Korean history. The male protagonist, Lee Kang Do, was among the survivors when he was a teenager. Now, as a young adult, he shows us symptoms of PTSD daily. He has constant flashbacks of being buried under the rubble with his leg pinned and witnessing someone dying. The flashbacks are dramatic and make him hyper-vigilant, so he is always on the lookout for possible threats and harm coming his way. These are all signs of PTSD. His flashbacks also trigger debilitating panic attacks.

Substance use as a means of coping is another aspect of PTSD. Since the tragedy, Kang Do has struggled with physical leg pain and gets by on painkillers. And the mall collapse destroyed Kang Do's chances of a soccer career, so he has become a down-and-out, bitter young adult who gets in street fights and cannot hold down a job. Yet he has a heart of gold—a classic K-Drama character trait. His life takes a positive turn when he meets the female protagonist, Ha Moon Soo, also a survivor of the mall collapse. Unlike Kang Do, she has been able to work through the PTS, even though she still has a phobia of elevators due to the trauma. However, it doesn't hamper her daily functioning as Kang Do's symptoms do, though it puts a damper on her quality of life since she prefers to walk flights of stairs.

What Rain or Shine does very well is display these PTSD symptoms clearly enough to identify in a systematic way. I can point them out to people without having to expose a real-life client. This is really a unique way to explain textbook symptoms of PTSD to teach people about this mental health disorder and encourage them or their loved ones get the help they need. Using the visuals is more effective than simply describing symptoms; as a clinician, it's very helpful to show what symptoms actually look like so clients see for themselves how they can manifest. It's validating to observe symptoms in someone that are otherwise uncomfortable to experience personally.

Kang Do's symptoms are both physical and mental. Of course, kudos to the actors (as always) for portraying such physical and emotional expressions. Throughout the K-Drama, we see Kang Do in anguish as he suffers with leg pain, both real and imagined, which is not uncommon with PTSD. The pain can feel more intense when one is triggered, experiencing the trauma as if they are living through it again, and then feeling the pain through that flashback. But seeing someone else having this kind of experience provides an externalization experience and helps distract from the "woe is me" mentality. Or, in some sense, misery loves company. It also takes away the loneliness, which is one of the very hardest aspects of dealing with mental illness and mental health conditions.

It's Okay to Not Be Okay (IOTNBO), 2020

Premiering on Netflix right at the start of the pandemic in March 2020, this hit K-Drama made a global mark. (Timing is everything.) This popular K-Drama is notable for the progressive way it features mental health conditions as well as mental illness. The lead characters, including one who has autism, have experienced childhood trauma and each of their stories centers on how they're navigating the trauma as adults. What's most interesting is that the story is set at a mental institution. For me, the best part was how it promoted more conversations around mental health in places and among people who weren't talking about it before.

IOTNBO showcases childhood trauma in the lead characters, with the female lead, Ko Moon Young, showing symptoms of PTSD years later. However, the main reason I talk about this K-Drama in many of my workshops and sessions is that it introduced what I would call an advanced technique used to treat trauma, particularly PTSD.

Episode two shows us the butterfly hug, a coping technique from the therapy known as Eye Movement Desensitization and Reprocessing (EMDR), which is used to alleviate distress associated with traumatic memories. EMDR, which requires extensive training for clinicians, is an evidence-based psychotherapy to help people recover from PTSD symptoms as well as disorders like anxiety, depression, and OCD. As you can imagine, it is surprising to see an EMDR method in any medium, let alone a K-Drama. I recognized it right away since I have training in EMDR. The episode shows Kim Soo Hyun's character, Moon Kang Tae, calming a distressed, angry Ko Moon Young by walking her through the butterfly hug. It's a way to self-soothe (known as desensitization in EMDR) through bilateral stimulation (like eye movement or tapping) to help process trauma. We see the female lead doing this, as well as Kang Tae's brother, Moon Sang Tae. For many clients and followers, *IOTNBO* was their gateway K-Drama. With its high-quality production and intelligent presentation of mental health conditions and mental illness, it's a good way to get engrossed in K-Dramas.

This show was a catalyst for conversations surrounding mental health and stigma and continues to have quite an impact today. Many folks tell me that *IOTNBO* inspired them to watch more K-Dramas because its compelling storytelling is informative and destigmatizing about mental health and mental illness. However, some people have also told me that its darker tone made it difficult to watch and they thought some of the scenes were too graphic. Overall, *IOTNBO* gained global recognition because of its progressive portrayal of mental health and mental illness, which until that point was barely discussed or recognized in Korean culture. It spurred conversation, questioning, and an unsettled feeling that can spur viewers to become more introspective, and to want to learn more.

The Glory, 2023

We can learn from *The Glory*, but not in the way you might think. It's almost reverse psychology. This K-Drama was a hot topic, and many people watched out of sheer curiosity and to avoid FOMO (fear of missing out). The main messages were about bullying, sexual harassment, and revenge, which are highly sensitive topics. As they say in journalism, if it bleeds, it leads—it's more exciting to talk about the scary stuff. The show was very well received in Korea because it highlighted the societal issue of bullying in Korea in such a drastic way. I am pleased that it promoted serious conversations on tackling bullying in Korea and admitting it was an acute systemic issue, one that can cause post-traumatic stress and PTSD, which is important for people to understand.

Research indicates that up to 20% of children in the United States ages 12–18 are bullying victims, which is a high number. However, it's important to point out misconceptions on what can cause PTSD. It's often assumed that PTSD comes only from something life-threatening, like a natural disaster, war, or being in a car accident. But researchers have found that childhood bullying can cause adult symptoms of PTSD and leave deep psychological scars. A study in *Child and Adolescent Psychiatry and Mental Health* indicates that among children who experienced bullying at school, 50% showed signs of PTSD.

In the first episode of *The Glory*, the female protagonist Moon Dong Eun is brutally bullied, and the flashbacks from her perspective throughout other episodes highlight her PTSD symptoms. *The Glory* was written by famed K-Drama writer Kim Eun Sook, which is initially why I watched it, but it is not one I recommend for uplifting viewing. However, I am discussing it here because it is instructional to analyze the idea that Moon Dong Eun's PTSD stems from her childhood trauma of being bullied throughout high school. While it may look like she is living her life well enough, functioning on a daily basis, her main purpose in life is seeking revenge for what happened to her. Some would say it's her way of healing from the unjustness done to her, and that the Han is what has kept her going all these years. However, in some sense, Dong Eun is disassociated from reality. She is far from healed, and I believe we are just seeing her healing begin at the end of the final episode. In an imagined K-Drama episode 17 (following the finale), we would see Moon Dong Eun seeking therapy to address her PTSD symptoms.

While revenge makes for thrilling drama, in and of itself revenge induces a vicious cycle of anger and hate. Although certainly understandable in light of the horrors like those Dong Eun endures at the hands of her merciless bullies, once you follow through with your revenge, where does that leave you? It may be satisfying to "win" in the end, but (spoiler alert) it leaves Dong Eun without meaning in her life, as we see at the end of *The Glory*. After all her bullies get their comeuppance, Dong Eun is about to die of suicide before someone stops her.

Many of my clients and followers have told me they couldn't get past the first or second episode because it was too triggering. Others have shared that they quite enjoyed *The Glory*, and were even empowered by Dong Eun's story, seeing her survive horrific trauma and get revenge on those who wronged her. But it's important to note that indulging in hateful emotions, no matter how terrible the trauma, isn't the answer to help the mental health healing process. What I would have preferred for her best revenge strategy would've been to rule the world and be successful in her career and personal life. (See the discussion about YouTuber Kwak Joon Bin below for more on this idea.)

So *The Glory* is not on my list of K-Dramas recommended for mental health. While it does highlight the subject in a way that can provide anti-bullying education, I found that many clients and followers couldn't watch due to the graphic scenes. While it was airing, I was often asked whether they should watch it. My response was that if anyone is hesitant to watch a certain K-Drama because they feel it will be distressing, that's their noonchi giving them the message that it's better to air on the side of caution and avoid watching it.

It's important to note what research tells us about watching graphic violence when it comes to PTSD. Not all the research is negative, meaning that it can be stimulating and provide a boost of adrenaline. Similarly, for those whose PTSD symptoms stem from military experience, watching combat scenes can provide a sense of comfort because it's familiar and helps validate their own experience. Those of my followers who watched *D.P. (Deserter Pursuit)* and served in the military also emphasized this. One of them commented, "It was oddly calming to watch D.P., even though it's not easy to watch. I enjoyed it a lot and it's one of my favorite K-Dramas because I really relate to the characters." (D.P. is also on my list of K-Dramas not necessarily recommended, but I did find well done.)

I'd like to end this chapter by sharing a story about a famous Korean travel YouTuber named Kwak Joon Bin. Last year, he revealed on the popular Korean talk show *You Quiz on the Block* that he was bullied throughout high school. His reveal came out just around the time *The Glory* had been released. Kwak Joon Bin explained that after high school, he ended up staying in his room for a couple of years, suffering from depression. At the point of considering suicide, he decided that wouldn't be fair for him to let the bullying get the better of him. He decided his best form of revenge would be to become as successful as possible. During the time he was holed up in his room, what cheered him up was watching travel shows and dreaming that he could someday travel around the world.

I loved his message to other victims of bullying: he realized he had been blaming himself for being bullied and decided that should not be the case, and wanted other bullying victims to know that they are not to blame for being bullied. As a therapist, I know that this is a key part of therapy and recovering from PTSD caused by bullying. I am proud and happy to see that Kwak Joon Bin has turned his trauma into a beautiful success story. Today, his YouTube Channel, KwakTube, has nearly two million subscribers and he's been traveling the world with well-known Korean celebrities. It doesn't come without wear and tear; he still has scars from the bullying, as anyone would. But he didn't let hate or anger overtake his decision-making. Instead, he chose to seek and define his own success and live to the best of his ability for his own sake. This is what is healthy for one's mental health.

K-Dramas That Accurately Portray PTSD:

- *The Glory*
- *Rain or Shine*
- *It's Okay to Not Be Okay*
- *Hometown Cha-Cha-Cha*
- *Chocolate*
- *D.P. (Deserter Pursuit)*

7 | K-Dramas and Suicide Awareness

South Korea has the number one suicide rate among OECD (Organization for Economic Co-Operation and Development) countries. It's held the highest suicide rate for almost 20 years, more than double the average for OECD member nations. Suicide has been a mainstay in K-Dramas for years. If you watch the older dramas from the 1990s into the 2000s, there's always a reference to a suicide in some form. Westerners have indicated they think the earlier K-Dramas, even as recently as five years ago, took suicide too lightly, seeming to downplay it or treat it inappropriately, almost as "commonplace." Some of this dislike stems from the fact that a character's suicide often wasn't highlighted or even talked about; it was just a part of the narrative.

It's important to recognize that cultural perspectives, traditions, and heritage influence attitudes toward suicide. The Korean perspective on what drives someone to suicide stems from the fact that the culture is rooted in Confucianism, which promotes peace, harmony, and collectivism. Historically, Koreans have used suicide to preserve that Confucian concept of peace and harmony because that is what is ingrained in society, what they have been educated to do for centuries. According to its epidemiology, suicide has been used as a badge of honor to protect the family's reputation and preserve its name. If you look at Korean history, leaders have died by suicide to avoid bringing shame to their families or the kingdom, to be seen as a martyr, or to show their honor by killing themselves for the sake of tradition and country. While this a part of Korea's history, it is by no means a healthy perspective. Speaking as a Korean American who's unbelievably proud of my culture and heritage, I disagree when historians or professors try to explain the high suicide rates in Korea today by bringing up the idea that suicide was seen as a badge of honor. We really need to explore the hidden or underlying conditions behind suicide, not simply dismiss the subject because of its historic context.

Jealousy, 1992

In Chapter 2, I explained how the 1992 K-Drama *Jealousy* changed my life when I was 18 years old. The lead, played by Choi Jin Sil, really resonated with me, and I grew to adore the actress because of the spunky and cute characters she portrayed. *Jealousy* was also the first K-Drama I watched to show a modern outlook on Korea, a country that was foreign to me at the time. Choi Jin Sil's acting and energy lured me in, and I looked up to her even though she was only seven years older than me. In fact, I cannot recall anyone else that I admire like I did Choi Jin Sil.

So you can imagine how devastated I was to hear of her suicide on October 2, 2008. Without knowing too much about the events surrounding her death, I just assumed she had succumbed to the pressures of Korean society, which would have been tremendous on a top Korean actress in her heyday who was even bigger in Korea than Julia Roberts was in the United States. That is, until she got divorced and became a single mother, which at that time was like walking around with a scarlet letter, because of those Confucian values embedded in Korean society. I had heard about her personal life, but I loved her for her character portrayals and didn't imagine the gossip, stigma, and career slowdown would impact her in the way it did.

She died by hanging herself. It's still so sad for me and resonates to this day because this is my field of work. I can imagine the stigma she must have faced in what is still considered a conservative society where being a single mother was "like having a personality disorder," according to Park Soo Na, a national entertainment columnist. I shudder as I write this because of this crude correlation to mental health. There was speculation that Choi died by suicide due to the distress and depression from the hate she received in relation to some financial scandal involving a male actor, as well as her being made a pariah as a divorced, single mother. Knowing the culture that still exists today, she most likely felt ashamed due to high society's standards of representing the traditional family person, and that may have led to a possible depression.

This leads me to explore how suicide is presented in today's K-Dramas. Three K-Dramas in the last few years have been particularly useful in my work in this area. They show examples of suicidality, which is an important aspect of my work in grief and trauma. This term, from the American Psychological Association, refers to suicidal ideation, making suicide plans, and attempting suicide. Each of these three K-Dramas shows a multidimensional look at suicide, which nevertheless only skims the surface about what leads people to end their life. I have seen that suicide leaves a permanent mark on the loved ones the deceased leaves behind: the experience of things left unresolved, the various "whys" of what led to a suicide, and then the guilt, regret, and sorrow that people must navigate as they wonder what it looks like to move on post-suicide and the stigma that comes with it.

The third episode of 2022's *Extraordinary Attorney Woo*, a stellar K-Drama that was popular globally, showed the parents of a son who died by suicide try to keep his suicide a secret. They indicated that they never wanted people to find out about their son's suicide. I believe the way *Extraordinary Attorney Woo* showcased social issues in Korean society is very telling of how suicide is handled in Korean society. However, I think the parents' decision in this K-Drama isn't uncommon since there exists such a high social stigma surrounding suicide everywhere, in all communities and societies. For instance, one of my followers, a white American nicknamed CJ living in the Pacific Northwest, shared that her nephew died of suicide more than 10 years earlier, and her sister has never talked about it to this day. Her nephew's death was never mentioned again, and she respectfully gives her sister space while she grieves in her own way. From my experience in working with families impacted by suicide, the silence over what happened and the need for private grieving are a common response.

Tomorrow, 2022

Tomorrow is a K-Drama that I hadn't expected to enjoy so much. This was the first K-Drama I chose to watch based solely on what my followers and clients were saying about it. It did put me in a dark place while I was watching, and my mood was somber throughout the viewing experience. I had expected that, which is why I was hesitant to watch it in the first place. The main storylines of *Tomorrow* concern suicidality. Every episode or two had a different story about the who, what, why, and how surrounding a character's decision to end their life. That was very effective storytelling in presenting the very varied reasons, circumstances, and situations behind a person's decision to end their life. For instance, the first two episodes involve a character bullied throughout high school, and her PTS symptoms return in full force in adulthood when she realizes the perpetrator has become famous for writing a book intended to comfort bullying victims. In episode six, we see that a Korean War veteran, who has struggled to have a thriving family and career life and feels his life is useless because of PTSD, has been having suicidal thoughts and has created a plan for suicide. Both of these situations are quite different reasons for contemplating suicide and making plans to end their life. The *Tomorrow* crisis management team gives them hope in a unique way, catering to both their mental health needs. And there are many moving stories in the other episodes in this K-Drama.

I appreciate that *Tomorrow* shows that suicide is not caused just by mental illness. In a sense, it teaches us that we are not immune to dying by suicide, because any life event can get us into an emotionally hopeless place where suicide may seem to be the answer. Hope is again the key word here. In each episode, the grim reapers "saved" someone from dying by suicide by providing them hope that they are not alone. This message is specifically why I use *Tomorrow* in my work. The grim reapers sought out each character who was on the brink of suicide, realizing what got them to that point of hopelessness.

As I share in my work, the grim reapers can be examples we glean from to help someone through their darkest of moments where they believe suicide is the answer. The grim reapers do not present them with a slew of solutions or even show them a glimpse of their life if they did something differently. What they do is what I do in my work as a therapist. It's what I call the trade secret of therapy and I always share it with my audience. The grim reapers in *Tomorrow* make the characters feel like they are not alone by validating what they're going through and giving them hope through their support.

Suicide is preventable, which is why we have suicide hotlines in the United States, and why even Korea has hotline numbers pasted on bridges where suicides tend to happen. In the dark moments of loneliness, reaching out to someone or having someone to talk to and share with is what can save lives. Again, the grim reapers in *Tomorrow* don't rush to save someone from suicide with a plan on how they can change their life. They approach them in empathy and compassion, knowing what drove them to that point, and give them hope by just being there. That's the trade secret of therapy.

"How could they do this? That's so selfish of them." Many clients impacted by suicide have told me they were angry at what they referred to as a "selfish decision." I've had physicians speak with me about how upset they were that a patient died by suicide and felt it was terribly selfish of them to do so. Because I'm in the position to hear many different sides of a story, I had never seen suicide as selfish because I understood from my own experience as well as through that of my clients that selfishness does not even come into play when one decides to end their life. People have pointed out to me that *Tomorrow*'s portrayal of suicide and the numerous reasons behind it gave them an empathy they did not previously have, realizing that suicide is so much more complex than they first believed. Folks have shared with me that the K-Dramas validated the understanding that the subject of suicide has many layers, and that is why it's difficult.

Taxi Driver, 2021

Taxi Driver offers a different spin on suicide in a dramatic storytelling fashion. The stable of main characters is known as the Rainbow Taxi Company, which is a cover for their vigilante justice. As a team working together, they provide "revenge" in the form of solutions for those wronged victims driven to such despair that they think suicide is their only option out of a distraught life. Although I'm not promoting revenge at all (far from it), the main message that we can take from *Taxi Driver* is similar to that of *Tomorrow*. The Rainbow Taxi Team gives the hopeless hope for a better life, because they showed they were in their corner fighting for them.

Suicidal ideation is extremely hard to talk about. Although research indicates it's not a definitive risk factor that leads to suicide, it is still a risk factor. In my work with the Asian American community, I have found that suicidal ideation is more common than not, due to the stressful expectations in the culture. At least 60% of the clients I've worked with have indicated suicidal ideation at some point in their life, including me when I was 14 years old. Based on my clinical experience and my own personal experience, suicidal ideation is exacerbated when you're lonely. Making suicide plans can empower you because you feel like you're taking control of your life. The Rainbow Taxi Company provided the empowerment in those critical moments. As they're about to end their life, the characters see their business card or sticker on the bridge, reading, for instance, "Don't kill yourself. Take revenge. We'll do it for you." The key phrase here is "for you."

Based on the numerous direct messages I received through my social media talking about *Taxi Driver* and *Tomorrow* the last few years, the portrayals of suicide in both of these series have been helpful for my clients and followers. Some of them shared that these K-Dramas "validated their experiences" when they were feeling suicidal. Others indicated that they're struggling with loneliness, but watching the

K-Dramas helps them feel like they aren't alone in this world and they're able to manage suicidal thoughts seeing the hope in these K-Drama stories.

True Beauty, 2021

True Beauty is a beauty of a K-Drama showing viewers how to navigate the aftereffects of suicide. Two high school friends have lost their friend to suicide, and both deal with it in different ways. Suicide was not necessarily a main part of the story, but it was an integral aspect of their estranged relationship. In episodes 11–12, the male protagonist finally admits he was wracked with guilt over their friend's suicide, and there ensues a conversation I find to be an effective way to understand how to navigate suicide for the loved ones to learn from. The character Lee Suho shares that he missed calls from their friend on the day of his suicide and Lee Suho feels that he should've been there for him. His estranged best friend, Han Seo Jun, is touched; it's the first he's heard of this and he hadn't realized how much his friend was grieving, as he himself was. This was their breakthrough—both finally understood that they had always been on the same page. I point out these two episodes as a very sensitive teaching moment, a catalyst for post-suicide healing to begin. CJ, one of my dedicated followers, told me that *True Beauty*'s example was healing for her; it was beneficial for her to see such a portrayal. Even though it was not the way her family members had handled the suicides of her stepfather and her maternal grandfather, she nevertheless saw it as a hopeful way of moving forward in her family's narrative of suicide, as well as for others who may have experienced a loved one's death by suicide.

One other important point is that a reason why suicide can be so shocking is that right before the suicide, the deceased might have seemed "fine" or "happy" after going through a "rough spell." In my work, I have seen this to be a tricky time because their mind may be clearer to formulate a suicide plan that they will carry out because they came out of rock bottom and don't want to experience it again. It is generally in a moment of clarity that suicide is carried out, as we see in the K-Dramas I'm talking about. This critical moment is quite emotional, but in that moment is where the grim reapers of *Tomorrow* come and "save" their lives by being there for them and with them.

All these K-Dramas bring a greater understanding of the why behind suicide. A former client of mine died of suicide the week of Thanksgiving several years ago. I had treated his wife before she met him, and after he came into her life, I saw them together as a couple. I discharged them a few months before their wedding and then the pandemic hit a few months later. One of her friends, a former colleague of mine, informed me of my former client's husband's suicide, which shocked me. I hadn't seen them in a while and kept thinking to myself, what happened? He was so happy at his wedding. A medical provider colleague who had also treated him said something that bothered me: that it was selfish of him, and how could he leave his wife and three stepchildren behind? As a therapist studying suicidality, I understood that suicide could be the least selfish decision the deceased makes before ending their life.

K-Dramas Highlighting Suicide Awareness:
- *Start-Up* (ep. 14)
- *Hometown Cha-Cha-Cha* (eps. 14, 15)
- *Be Melodramatic* (eps. 1, 9)
- *True Beauty* (eps. 11, 12)
- *Tomorrow* (main theme)
- *Taxi Driver* 1 (main theme)

8

K-Dramas
and Coping
with Depression

"I am so thankful my children and nephews introduced me to watching K-Dramas. They teach me life lessons on how to handle my problems, depression, and how to love."

Depression is, well, depressing. One of the many things I say about depression is to understand that depressed people do not necessarily look depressed. It is a misconception that when you're depressed, you walk around moping like Eeyore in *Winnie the Pooh* and it is obvious to everyone. Not true, according to my experience with clients and the DSM (The Diagnostic and Statistical Manual of Mental Illnesses), our diagnosis manual. I often see depression in the form of anger (such as Han), frustration, irritability, and lashing out, particularly in the Asian population. Also, depressed people may try hard to appear happy for the sake of others, so they put on a "happy face." This is why depression can be difficult to diagnose even though it is one of the most common mental health conditions. It is also why it can be a shock when someone dies by suicide, especially when they just saw the person looking happy.

Although depression is a common mental health condition and disorder, it is very much misunderstood. In my sessions with clients, I have found depression to be the toughest condition to explain to family members. For a family therapist, it is key in therapy for the identified client to have a strong support system, so I am constantly educating family members about what the client is going through and how to help. It is a collaborative process. Although they don't mean to be dismissive, family members often ask their loved one, "There's so much to be happy about. Why can't you just be happy?" What that ends up doing is sending their loved ones (my clients) into a tailspin of doubt, guilt, and shame.

Bringing K-Dramas into group sessions and workshops came about early in the pandemic to cheer people up because many folks were depressed and anxious amid a global lockdown. I kept saying that a global lockdown would make anyone depressed, meaning that depression can be normal in times of crisis and adversity. At any given time, we can feel depressed, but this does not mean we have depression. Yet a prolonged state of feeling depressed, if unresolved or not managed well, can later become depression and be diagnosed as such. I am seeing this more and more, even as we have emerged from the pandemic. Depression is also fairly prominent in K-Dramas, but I have narrowed it down to three examples.

Crash Landing on You, 2019

Yoon Seri is a beautiful and smart CEO, covering up a sad, lonely girl who wants to be loved by her stepmother and family and have other fulfilling relationships. When we are first introduced to her, we see her running a successful beauty company, coming from a *chaebol* (corporate conglomerate) family. However, as her story unfolds, we learn that she is disconnected from her family and disengaged with her stepmother through no fault of her own. Here's a reminder that depressed people don't necaessarily look depressed. On the outside, Yoon Seri appears happy, confident, and strong. In fact, one would be envious of all that she seems to have. This is a familiar story; a number of high-profile celebrities have revealed that they suffer from depression, and in some shocking cases, celebrities have died by suicide when no one saw it coming because they were what would be described as "on top of the world." In one of the story flashbacks, we see Yoon Seri lost in her thoughts in Switzerland, preparing to jump off a bridge to end her life. She records a message (a farewell note), and she never gets to jump because she's saved by her future love interest, who asks her to take a photo of him and his then fiancée.

I'm pointing this out because depression is that confusing and complex. It's such a miserable feeling that people work so hard to make themselves happy that they invalidate their emotions, which ends up exacerbating their symptoms. Yoon Seri's story resonated with many Asian Americans who face high expectations based on cultural norms in their communities and families. One of my followers said she cried for days after watching the scene where Yoon Seri tells her stepmother incredulously that it's her dream to be doing what she is doing, and her stepmother responds with disgust and rebukes her for being a CEO of her own company and not being part of the family business. The stepmother declares, "How dare you think of your own dream?" My follower, who's an Asian American female from the Northeast, felt Seri's pain since that was her situation just a few years prior when she told her parents that her dream was not to follow the path they designed for her but to quit her corporate job and move abroad and be involved in the creative arts. This young woman says she felt so suffocated that she fell into a depression and sought help, which included medication. This is a familiar scenario, which is why we were all so happy watching Yoon Seri and her stepmother have a breakthrough following the stepmother's reveal that she had been suffering from depression. Remember, in the end, managing depression is very much dependent on your support system.

My Liberation Notes, 2022

"Why is it so hard being sober?" The female protagonist asks her love interest, Mr. Gu, this pointed question. This K-Drama was on my favorites list in 2022. It's written by the same writer of *My Mister* (which I'll discuss later in the chapter), which is one of my all-time favorites. Mr. Gu (Gu sshi in Korean) is fascinating. He is depressed, wracked by guilt from the death of his former girlfriend, and burdened by the toll of his work in the underground world. Mr. Gu copes by abusing alcohol, to numb his emotions and thoughts, and to avoid his past demons. Research has shown that there appears to be a bidirectional relationship between depression and alcohol use. Both issues are among the most prevalent psychiatric disorders and co-occur often.

Mr. Gu is also the epitome of the Eeyores we imagine walking about moping and with sullen expressions. Research shows that depression and substance abuse often coexist. Depression is hard, and coping with it by managing your symptoms takes daily persistence and diligence. It is "exhausting being sober" as Mr. Gu points out in episode 16, when Mi Jeong, his love interest, asks him why he drinks from morning until night. He admits that when he's sober, the people from his past come to him, approaching him to face things and he hears all these voices, so it's easier to drink to wipe it all away.

Mi Jeong's response is beautiful and one that I point out to clients as the most likely changing point for Gu sshi. What can we take away from her response? Perhaps to find a way to be like that in our own lives for someone we know who is suffering from depression. It's no surprise that depression is exacerbated (as many mental health conditions are) by feeling judged or misunderstood for experiencing what we are experiencing. It's the nature of our brain to err on the side of judgmental and be negative. Our first response to Mr. Gu in real life most likely would've been about what we can do to help him stop drinking, or to suggest he get rehab treatment. Instead, Mi Jeong doesn't offer solutions. She takes an approach that lets her relate in her own way, validating the very demons behind why Mr. Gu drinks. What I think is profound is that she states she isn't an alcoholic (pointing out that Gu sshi is), but she also has those demons and struggles with hearing voices. This is our takeaway. Solutions can always come, and we can figure them out together. But what a person needs most is to feel like they're understood even in their worst moment. Again, it's the trade secret of therapy.

What I find most interesting, based on client and follower feedback, was how popular Mr. Gu was. Of course, it had a lot to do with him being mysteriously sexy, which is always alluring for viewers. However, many folks found his vulnerability and depressed character just as appealing. We don't necessarily have to be going through something like the character is to empathize and cheer them on; they want to see them happy. This is generally the case for all of us when we're watching K-Dramas, especially when we see characters struggling. This example provides me with a good form of reference when I am asking the people who make up the depressed client's support system to understand what their loved one is going through. We tend to be more compassionate for depressed K-Drama characters than we show in real life to our depressed loved ones, whom we want to feel better immediately because it's easier for us. Let's face it, no one wants to be around a depressed person. It's a downer. Let's use this example from Mi Jeong as a takeaway of connecting with our loved ones with depression so they can find the strength to get better.

Gu sshi changed on his own, not because Mi Jeong made him change. He felt loved and seen by her and it gave him the courage to make changes in his life toward getting sober. I want to be clear that, despite the happy ending we see in *My Liberation Notes*, Gu sshi still has a long way of healing and sobering ahead of him. That's the assumption we must conclude, but he is on the road to recovery in many ways by the K-Drama's end.

Reply 1988, 2015

To date, this is the only K-Drama that comes to mind showing female characters experiencing the emotional turmoil of menopause, as well as talking about it with one another. In episode 19, the three main mothers of the drama, Ra Miran (Jung Hwan's mother), Lee Il Hwa (Deok Sun's mother), and Kim Sun Young (Sunwoo's mother) talk about feeling depressed through menopause, which is an effective way to navigate a normal but emotionally tumultuous life stage. Menopause is a natural process that causes physical and mental symptoms and, speaking from my experience as a therapist, it is one of the toughest life stages for women. Treatment methods include estrogen therapy (hormones), antidepressants, and lifestyle changes, which is an indicator of what goes on during menopause. Studies show that women going through menopause are at one and a half to three times increased risk of major depression.

We see it in *Reply 1988*, especially through the eyes of one of the mothers, Ra Miran. She has trouble sleeping and eating, will cry at the drop of a hat for no particular reason, and sits on the sofa in a catatonic state. She also struggles with simple tasks such as cooking or housework that she has been used to doing daily. These are all symptoms specific to depression (among other conditions). *Reply 1988* provides psychoeducation surrounding the perimenopausal stage, which I think is impactful, and I absolutely love how it's done. Ra Miran shares with her family how they can help her and what she will be experiencing as she goes through menopause. This is a terrific teaching moment and a therapist's dream. It's important to be able to share your needs, indicate how your support system can meet them, and ask for help when you need it. For a drama showing Asian culture, I was blown away by this scene because it's been such a stigma in our community to ask for help, discuss our depressed feelings, and state what we want to see happen that will help us.

Go ahead and bookmark episode 19 of *Reply 1988* right now. Ra Miran invites her family to engage in her menopause "treatment," and here's where the family's response is critical. As a family therapist, I always look at the overall family system. The family's response to a client's depression, whether it's situational or clinical (long-term), can aid the client's healing in a tremendous way. I have seen it and cannot emphasize this enough. There's a poignant scene where the oldest son, after hearing his mother out and being very enthusiastic about helping her around the house, calls his younger brother, who's out of town working as an officer in the army. He tells him to call their mother as often as he can to keep her spirits lifted since she misses him. What a wonderful follow-up by the son.

Reply 1988 is the first K-Drama I recommended in a therapy session years ago and the rest is history, so this is a special one to me. But it's also a special one to many. In fact, I still get surprised seeing how many people of all ages adore *Reply 1988*, from Gen Zs to baby boomers like my parents. If there's a K-Drama to connect people around the world, this is it. I love reading the responses from followers who have a common theme, and that relates to how *Reply 1988* brought them closer to their parents. One woman shared how seeing this menopause episode taught her how to be a better daughter to her mother in menopause because she underestimated its impact. Another person told me that he hadn't realized his mother was depressed until watching *Reply 1988*. He saw his mother in all the mothers in the K-Drama and came to an understanding that she needed to feel needed. This was something he didn't communicate to his mother over a period of many years. He told me he's watched *Reply 1988* many times and learns something new each time, and he finds another way to show his mother how much he appreciates her. He feels closer to her now than he ever did.

Our Blues, 2022

For me, *Our Blues* was the first K-Drama that provides an explanation and shows what clinical depression looks like through the character Min Seon-Ah. To be honest, I was quite surprised to see such an excellent portrayal and immediately included her character development in my work. Clinical depression is a persistent depression (even lifelong), and it's more severe than the depression caused by grief or menopause. Clinical depression can affect people of any age, including children. From my experience, and from what the research indicates, clinical depression symptoms can improve with both therapy and medication working in tandem. This is what we see in *Our Blues* with the character Seon-Ah. When we first encounter her, she's lying in bed drenched in water or sweat, symbolizing the heaviness she feels, being drowned in her sorrows.

When we're first getting to know Seon-Ah, we see her struggling to manage basic hygiene. Her husband, who doesn't hide his frustration, tells her to take care of herself better, telling her she needs a shower because she's starting to smell. He's also snapping at her to find the will to live. This is a typical reaction from family members. Later on, Seon-Ah's husband comes home with their son after dark because she completely lost track of time and forgot to pick him up from school. Seon-Ah and her husband end up divorcing and he takes full custody of their son, which devastates her.

My clients have described clinical depression as walking around with a dark cloud hovering over you constantly. The dark cloud creates a fog where you cannot see clearly, so you're driving or walking slowly because you don't know where you're going. They also indicate that the fog sometimes makes it hard to breathe so they're sluggish. Clients have told me there are moments they feel like they see the sun peeking out, but when they try to get some sunshine, the clouds take over and the sun disappears, so they stop trying to find the sun. We're able to visualize this in a way through the portrayal of Seon-Ah in *Our Blues*.

What I want people to take away from Seon-Ah is the progression of her growth and healing, as we see her navigating clinical depression. Several things show us that she is working hard in taking care of her depression: 1) She reveals the history of depression in family. Her father, who also suffered from depression, died by suicide before her eyes by driving his car into the ocean. 2) She shares about her treatment and progress with Dong Seok, the man in love with her and with whom she later ends up. 3) We see Seon-Ah feeling better, working and living on her own to get back custody of her son and renovating a future house on Jeju Island. 4) We see her co-parenting well with her ex-husband, who also sees her progress, and therefore allows her more visits with their son.

The conversation between Seon-Ah and Dong Seok in episode 10 is a very good example of how loved ones can show their support. Dong Seok asks Seon-Ah questions about her depression, such as when it started, what her symptoms feel like, and what kind of help she is getting. He also asks pointedly, "Is it treatable?" to which Seon-Ah says, "According to my doctor, it is treatable." Asking questions is a wonderful way to connect with your loved one, inviting them to share what they're going through without the intervention of a therapist. It's what I encourage of my clients' support system. If you don't ask questions, how do you know how to help them? Seon-Ah also tells Dong Seok she is going to start therapy because she thinks she needs more than just medication. Research on clinical depression indicates both methods done conjointly is effective. Dong Seok's reaction is what I want you to learn from. He tells her all that sounds good and when she needs someone or is feeling depressed, she can call him.

Stigma surrounding therapy is one thing, but there's also a stigma against taking psychotropic medication. Some clients have told me they're fine taking medication and feel like it would help their therapy treatment but are hesitant because of negative reactions they anticipate from their family, including partner or spouse, older children, and siblings. In fact, many times that's a big reason why clients decide to stop taking medication or don't bother starting even though it is recommended as part of their treatment. For something like clinical depression, which is long-term, I have seen patients benefiting from taking psychotropic medication consistently while doing psychotherapy. Some have taken medication for decades and they're living well with clinical depression, though they fight through bouts here and there. As Seon-Ah says in *Our Blues,* quoting her doctor, depression (mental illness) is treatable.

A follower told me she was watching *Our Blues* with her family, and thanks to the character of Seon-Ah, she realized that the depression she had been experiencing off and on since she was a teen could be treatable if she pursued therapy, and possibly medication. This person indicated she had questioned for years whether she was depressed but didn't have the strength to find out more. She had resorted to thinking she would be miserable, and maybe sometimes not miserable, for the rest of her life. Watching Seon-Ah, and seeing her improve over time and be happy through this K-Drama, made this person realize she could be happy too, if she invested in treatment.

There are numerous stories like this, where folks tell me that K-Dramas have given them a window into their head and heart when it comes to their mental health. It always brings tears to my eyes, because watching a story like this from a K-Drama can change your life.

My Mister, 2018

From clients to followers to random strangers I meet who watch K-Dramas, many people tell me how much these shows cheer them up when they need it. Many K-Dramas fall into the romantic comedy genre and even include slapstick humor. People say that when they watch K-Dramas and laugh out loud, they forget they're sad. My Mister is one of those I recommend you watch to cheer you up, although it won't make you laugh out loud.

This one is my all-time favorite K-Drama. To put it bluntly, it is not a happy-go-lucky K-Drama. Initially, I didn't have a desire to watch until at least a couple years after it came out because it looks depressing and does not really draw you in when you read the synopsis. However, I had heard enough good things about it from several folks that I decided to try it on my own. Wow. It blew me away. So I tell people who struggle with depression to watch My Mister. although that doesn't mean My Mister will have the same impact on everyone, and some people are indeed skeptical about this recommendation.

This K-Drama is melancholy and somber with a beautiful silver lining of hope as its core theme. This silver lining is critical to the message of the story. I felt hopeful from the very first episode and it's my plea that others feel and see that as well when they watch this gem of a K-Drama. It's why I believe when you are feeling depressed or suffering from depression, My Mister gives you the hope you need for the strength required to pull you through your tough moment. You see, the lead characters are depressed. They're not suffering from depression per se, but they have the weight of the world on their shoulders, and both are experiencing a low point in their lives. The male protagonist is Park Dong Hoon, who's in a mid-life crisis, while Lee Jian, the female protagonist, is in a young adult crisis at the age of 21. They happen to work in the same company. As Jian narrates in the latter half of the K-Drama, she's at the bottom of the totem pole at work so no one pays attention to her. However, Park Dong Hoon takes notice of her aloneness one day and invites her out to a company dinner, which she says changes her life. Both are experiencing depressive symptoms and are not happy but find solace in their friendship. It's important to note that what makes this K-Drama especially poignant is the jeong between these two characters. There's nothing sexual about it; although Jian admits to having a crush on him because she so admired who he was, theirs was truly a friendship for the ages.

I suggest this drama for those suffering from depression or feeling depressed because *My Mister* takes you through the journey of two downtrodden people, which through the kindness and goodness of Park Dong Hoon ends in healing and happiness for Jian. What more could you want? We are watching a character (Jian) transform emotionally from depressed to hopeful. She is also transforming socially from distrusting and cynical to trusting and grateful. The transformation is complete in episode 16 (no spoilers here) when we see where life has taken her. Meanwhile, Park Dong Hoon finds transformation through his care for Jian, which leaves him with self-confidence and a renewed vigor that makes him feel successful and happy.

I'm not the only one who thinks so highly of this show. *My Mister* won the Korean Baeksang Art Award for best K-Drama in 2019. And nearly everyone who has watched *My Mister* absolutely loves it and sees the beauty in it. I just add a layer to it to help folks with their mental health, especially depression (but also anxiety). This K-Drama shows us not only a literal transformation in its characters, but we are also transformed by their transformation. This K-Drama can impact your life for the better.

K-Dramas Accurately Portraying Depression:

- *My Mister* (Park Dong Hoon)
- *My Liberation Notes* (Mr. Gu)
- *Vincenzo* (Jang Han Seo)
- *Crash Landing on You* (Yoon Seri)
- *Our Blues* (Kim Seona)
- *Our Beloved Summer* (Kook Yeon Soo)
- *Reply 1988* (Ra Miran)

9 | K-Dramas and Managing Anxiety

"If you can't stop watching K-Dramas, it's because they de-stress your distress. A dose of a K-Drama a day can help manage your anxiety that can lead you astray."

This is one of my anecdotes that went viral, and I received a lot of responses. I've said I watch K-Dramas for my own self-care, and I believe most K-Drama viewers de-stress their distress this way. Anxiety can lead you astray if you are not proactively taking care of your stress on a daily basis. It's what I call mental health hygiene. We're very good at our physical hygiene, but that also needs to include mental health hygiene—the health of our mind.

Back in May 2021 I inadvertently tried an experiment. I didn't watch K-Dramas that entire month for two reasons: 1) I was very busy with virtual workshops, presentations, and keynotes since it was mental health month and AANHPI month. And 2) I simply didn't prioritize my mental health whatsoever. It was the longest I have ever gone without watching a K-Drama in recent years. Now that I look back, I'm not sure what I was thinking, but I know I was in survival mode. There was quite a demand for my speaking and my work with increased workplace anxiety, the spike in anti-Asian violence, including the Atlanta spa shooting tragedy. I was swamped and I strayed from my normal schedule by sidelining my self-care via K-Dramas.

Instead, I prioritized my career and added as many virtual events to fill my schedule as best I could (everything was still in lockdown then). It was an unprecedented time. I felt excitement and passion for my work. However, my mental health and physical health took a major hit. Because I ignored a flair-up with an inner ear condition (Ménière's disease), I lost a good amount of hearing in my left ear. Today I have a hearing aid and am living with moderate hearing loss. I am sharing this because K-Dramas didn't just relax me for the sake of stress management. K-Dramas also helped me stay in tune with my body in practicing muscle relaxation, which is part of the K-Drama viewing process, whether we know it or not. I believe I would've identified the ringing in my ear had I been practicing my self-care routine by watching a dose of a K-Drama a day, which helps my body to calm down.

De-stressing is what I have found to be the most common and popular response to watching K-Dramas. Someone sent me a message a couple of years ago talking about how he had struggled with panic attacks since he was a young adult. Although he was able to handle them, he was still fearful of them growing more frequent because he kept worrying that he would have panic attacks, which became a self-fulfilling prophecy. His partner told him about my work and how I use K-Dramas for mental health. He thought he could assign himself homework to watch a K-Drama to help him relax and distract him through a panic attack. He knew when he was about to experience one and they weren't so much debilitating as they were embarrassing, because he would have trouble breathing and needed to walk away and be by himself. When he messaged me, he mentioned how he first tried 2019's *Vagabond* because he likes action when he is distressed, but it didn't really help. However, he decided to try again and watch 2013's *Inheritors* when he had a panic attack at his partner's house, and it did the trick. He says that now when he thinks about watching K-Dramas for enjoyment, he can feel his body relaxing even before he turns one on.

What an amazing story. Although I know this won't work for everyone who struggles with panic attacks, I do think it's why many folks turn to K-Dramas—because they're soothing, and reading the subtitles (for the vast majority of viewers who aren't Korean) can be a welcome distraction from your thoughts. When your mind is calm (think mindfulness), it gives your body a chance to relax because you're breathing more effectively. I tell clients the purpose of deep breathing is really about science. It's to get oxygen to the brain, so it can function properly. When we are distressed, we're either holding our breath or hyperventilating. Through deep breathing techniques, our brain gets the oxygen it needs to work the way it should. Then it tells our muscles to relax, which in turn calms us down.

One of my gal pals of several years, Hiromi Okuyama, a content creator and actress I "met" on the audio app Clubhouse, recently fell in love with K-Dramas after hearing me tell her about them for quite a while. She has even moderated my K-Drama and mental health talks on Clubhouse, but that still didn't have her turn to K-Dramas until last year. She was initially of the mindset that many others share—that they do not have time for K-Dramas. You may think Hiromi would credit me for turning to K-Dramas in her time of distress, but it's not in the way you think.

Hiromi had been having some family struggles the last few years and turned to me for guidance and support when she needed a therapist and a friend. She had been seeing a psychologist, but felt it was a hassle at times to make an appointment. Unbeknownst to me, she had been feeling guilty for taking my time and decided to try to cope as best as she could without my help because she felt bad for bothering me. During a recent bout of struggles. she felt like she needed to take my advice and watch a K-Drama. Hiromi tells me she couldn't get past the guilt of bothering me (she was never a bother, I tell her) and felt like she had to turn to K-Dramas as a way of communicating with me and to help her through her tough time. Well, as you can imagine, she ended up not needing me after all because the first K-Drama she watched, *Hometown Cha-Cha-Cha,* did the trick. She shared this with me not necessarily to give me kudos, but to express her enthusiasm on how much K-Dramas are helping her, marveling at what they've provided in her life: respite from distress, an opportunity to learn more about herself, and a chance to be a better mother to her kids.

Hiromi says, "It was so sweet and loving. I find that many American shows are in your face, trying to be edgy, and push your boundaries. They're clickbait-y. But *Hometown Cha-Cha-Cha* felt so warm, and is so wholesome that it was comforting. I can see why people watch it to feel better." I think Hiromi sums it up nicely. To de-stress, we need to seek a level of comfortability in viewership.

Pandemic and Politics

Beyond the conditions of a global lockdown in early 2020, quite a few people in the United States also turned to K-Dramas because they were distressed over the tumultuous political climate. I know this all too well because, in my clinical work for companies and families, I was doing a lot of crisis management surrounding the contention during the fall of 2020. It was a time of extreme adversity, and everything was exacerbated by the stress surrounding Covid. People told me they found K-Dramas comforting and soothing and just what they needed. The more they watched them, the more they wanted to continue watching them, and as we say in K-Drama world, "there we go down the rabbit hole" into a whole new world that folks say has greatly enhanced their life. People have told me they wanted to be in Korea during the pandemic because as they were watching K-Dramas, they felt that they could trust Korea and its people. I found this interesting because it's an angle I hadn't really thought of until they shared about it. Several professionals on one of my coaching calls (it's always fun to talk K-Dramas in sessions when you least expect it) said that they found K-Dramas refreshing, especially for how wholesome they are. Again, in a time of Covid and U.S. political tensions, K-Dramas met their needs and they liked what they saw.

These conversations at the time really helped me on a personal level. It got me thinking about K-Dramas from a different angle. They were reflecting a society rooted in traditional norms that I struggled with and talk a lot about in my work today, and Americans appreciated that so much. Often, when one feels unsafe and distrusting of the environment in which they live, there's such anxiety that they seek "shelter" where they can find it. This is a coping mechanism, and it happened to come in the form of K-Dramas, which Americans especially welcomed with open arms because they were a pleasant distraction from the fraught environment. During a vulnerable time, Americans found Korean cultural traditions and values beautifully different, and interest piqued in the United States to learn more about South Korea.

Practicing Mindfulness

I have a slew of stories, especially from teachers, who noticed a spike in their anxiety during the pandemic. No surprise, since we all know how stressful things were during this vulnerable time, especially in the schools. Teachers of all races and ethnicities across the country have shared how much K-Dramas allow them time to decompress after a tough day working with students and dealing with anxious parents, particularly as we navigate mass shootings around the country. They've found K-Dramas comforting, a way to refuel after a taxing day with students who have been really struggling to adjust in a post-pandemic world.

The same goes for clinical and medical providers. Over the last three years I have seen more clinical colleagues on my social media who have come to understand why I use K-Dramas in my work. I was met with skepticism early on because colleagues didn't quite see the connection to mental health—or even to hear me out because it was completely out of the ordinary. However, I ignored the critics and hearsay and followed my noonchi with what made sense: to talk about mental health during the pandemic in a unique way, the "breath of fresh air" that Priscilla Kwon was talking about.

Things do look different today. More people in the providing professions seem to be turning to K-Dramas as their form of self-care. While it doesn't surprise me, it does make me giddy. This group isn't easy to win over, so now that it's happened there's a sense of satisfaction and, honestly, the credibility that a licensed professional looks for when it comes to evidence-based research. I love hearing from fellow therapists around the world who share their points of view on the K-Dramas I discuss on my platform. Many indicate it's a great form of mindfulness (as do client and followers) because they need to focus on subtitles in order to understand what's going on in the story, and therefore do not multitask. I have indicated that K-Dramas can be an effective form of mindfulness practice for that reason because it keeps you in the present moment to absorb peace and gratitude.

It's wonderful hearing that people are forming K-Drama clubs at work, which is also a terrific mindfulness practice, essential in the workplace in many ways. As an executive coach, I tend to hear professionals say that they're too busy for mindfulness. My response is that the busier you are, the more you need mindfulness. One of the participants on my September tour said that she discovered K-Dramas in 2022 and was immediately hooked, so she started looking for others to talk with about them. Imagine her surprise and excitement when she discovered fellow physicians in her practice who also watched K-Dramas. She told us on the tour that they now have a K-Drama physician self-care group.

Being a provider myself, I find that compassion fatigue (burnout) has been increasingly prevalent after the pandemic, and mindfulness is key to managing stress to prevent burnout. A terrific way to do this is to have a group like a K-Drama club at work (or other groups with shared interests), not only to feel connected but also to de-stress by holding conversations that are not about work. K-Drama stories do well for this because people are relating to the characters and stories and therefore able to practice externalization, which as I've mentioned before helps distance the issue we're dealing with apart from ourselves. Mindfulness is also about being nonjudgmental, being grounded with your emotions, thoughts, and sensations. When we're reflecting on the stories and characters in K-Dramas, we learn from examples of what they're going through or how they've overcome an obstacle in their life, which in turn provides us a way to observe ourselves in a distant manner that doesn't allow the judgment to come in. Being judgmental about what we're feeling and thinking doesn't help us and can exacerbate our stress because what we feel is what we feel. When we see the K-Drama characters we love judging themselves, many of us actually speak to them (you know, when you speak to the TV screen or your phone?), telling them not to be so hard on themselves. This in turn helps us realize we're being hard on ourselves, which shifts our perspective. I love seeing the light bulb going off when the mindfulness of K-Drama viewing brings about the realization of how we can change by learning from the stories and characters.

One important aspect of mindfulness is always to make sure that what you're watching isn't actually distressing you. Just because it's K-Drama and you adore them doesn't mean you need to watch all of them or that all of them are benefiting your well-being. Yes, I believe in K-Dramas for mental health, but knowing what stresses me out or what may be too intense for me, I am choosy about which ones I watch. While we all like different genres, there are K-Dramas out there that aren't necessarily beneficial for each person's mental health. The following K-Dramas are ones I found intriguing and interesting, but I do not believe they can help de-stress your distress:

- *Mask Girl*
- *D.P.*
- *The Glory*
- *Juvenile Justice*
- *Little Women*
- *My Name*
- *Squid Game*
- *Extracurricular*
- *Sky Castle*
- *Save Me*

However, there's a slew of K-Dramas that I recommend to boost your mood:

- *Mr. Queen*
- *Love to Hate You*
- *Splash Splash Love*
- *Hometown Cha-Cha-Cha*
- *Good Manager*
- *Welcome to Waikiki*
- *Strong Girl Bong Soon*
- *Business Proposal*
- *Shopping King Louie*
- *Extraordinary Attorney Woo*
- *King the Land*

> *"If you can't stop watching K-Dramas, it's because they serve a good balance of escapism and realism. A dose of a K-Drama a day is not about escaping your reality, but helping you live through it in your own authentic way."*

I'm often asked whether it's okay to watch K-Dramas to escape from the stressors of life, and as I've made clear before, the answer is yes. But let me expand on this by explaining more about anxiety. Anxiety is a normal part of the human experience, so it's natural to have it in your life during times of family crisis, a global health pandemic, job insecurity, when you're feeling ill, or any number of other stressful situations. I tell clients: "If we resist, it will persist." By this I mean that resisting by avoiding our stressors—which tends to be a common reaction in Asian culture—ends up making it worse. As I mentioned before, Asians tend to err on the side of avoidance because the culture is rooted in Confucianism and they don't want to ruffle feathers or cause conflict. This is why I tend to see Asian families with a high level of stress, because very little is being communicated. We also see this in our K-Dramas, where families do not talk directly about the conflict at hand and try to navigate through it silently. However, I cannot emphasize enough that facing conflict, while it may be very uncomfortable, or even terrible, is a way to turn things upside down for the sake of positive change and growth. You want to live your life to the fullest, and often what you watch in a K-Drama can provide life lessons for you to do that.

We *do* need escapism in our lives. It's a psychological strategy of coping. Escaping by watching TV (or any other medium) is helpful in distracting you from your problems in real life. K-Drama escapism can transport you into a faraway world where none of your own issues or conflicts exist. You also feel connected to the characters (actors) in the form of a parasocial relationship (a type of one-sided relationship where someone gives time, attention, and emotional energy to a celebrity or other well-known figure, who has no idea they exist). Escapism can be a helpful way of dealing with challenging problems, managing your stress for daily mental health hygiene, and regulating your emotions.

However, in the same breath, there needs to be a balance, and escaping from your own life (or reality) is not what I am talking about. If you find yourself watching K-Dramas to avoid feeling the negative emotions or avoid dealing with making decisions in your own life, and also letting your responsibilities slide such as your job or housework or parenting, then it's time to step back because you are watching too much. This is why I say, "a *dose* of a K-Drama a day," which equates to on average one K-Drama episode—a little over an hour a day. I also like to say that the "only drama in your life should be a K-Drama." Here are a few good indicators that you're using escapism in a healthy way:

You feel happier and more relaxed.
You feel more rested and have energy to follow through with your responsibilities.

You may still feel anxious about what you need to get done or who you need to face, but you still choose to follow through. You do not disconnect from your real-life relationships.

"K-Dramas are my refuge, a safe space for me to feel peace,"
—Noona's Noonchi follower

Out of all the questions I ask on my platform, I get the most responses whenever I ask a variation of "How have K-Dramas helped your mental health?" and many of these answers are quite reflective and insightful. I tend to ask this question every so often since it's the reason behind Noona's Noonchi. Nearly all responses refer to how K-Dramas provide comfort and give them the sense that "everything will be okay." Clients and followers have told me that K-Dramas help them escape from the harsh realities of life, albeit briefly, providing the respite they need to recover. I tend to hear that K-Dramas are people's reward after a long day at work or school. I can't think of a better way to end the day—I use K-Dramas for my own self-care, in moderation, of course.

K-Dramas aren't necessarily just to de-stress either. On my tours, we watched K-Drama episodes on the bus rides for the fun of it since we were headed to the K-Drama filming sites. A couple of the bus rides were at least three to five hours long, but participants told me the time flew by because they were enjoying K-Dramas. Because we were on vacation, I found myself telling everyone that binging five episodes of *Business Proposal* from Busan to Seoul was well worth it for the tour's sake. I am writing this with a chuckle because as a tour host, I was stressed about whether the tour participants would find the long bus rides grueling. However, thanks to *Business Proposal*, *Hometown Cha-Cha-Cha*, *When the Camellia Blooms*, and *Mr. Sunshine*, as well as BTS YouTube videos, by the time we reached Seoul on day seven of the tour they were relaxed, as was I.

The Powerful Intersectionality of K–Dramas and Identity

10 | K-Dramas and Life Stages

We are psychologically attached to our identity. It gives us belongingness, meaning, and purpose because our identity is rooted in our core values, world schemas, and cultural heritage. Our identity is ever evolving as we're experiencing various stages of life. There is a direct correlation between mental health and identity, which is why it's a large part of my work. As I mentioned before, what makes K-Dramas so effective is the depth of character development. The character's identity, depending on their season of life, is a huge draw for audiences because they're very relatable and events unfold in real time (K-Drama time). The flagship workshop in my Cultural Confidence® core series addresses how our mental health intersects with our identity. It's where I begin when I'm explaining my Cultural Confidence® model and defining mental health and identity, which is the foundation of our growth.

In fact, most of my clinical and coaching work centers on how we perceive ourselves, our values, our experiences, our background, and so on in order to understand our emotional, psychological, and social well-being. All these elements we see in our beloved K-Dramas. It's why we get so involved with the characters, because not only are we identifying with their emotions, but also with their identity crises at the time they're going through it. While there's a direct correlation between mental health and identity, I have found that the relationship to our own identity (i.e., having a strong self-identity, or struggling with self-identity) is what impacts our mental health. Regardless of what we are going through, how we feel in terms of belonging to our own self is what keeps us strong and steady. When we waiver in that and experience self-doubt, we can allow narratives to seep in that conflict with our core values. When we identify this in K-Dramas, we learn from it because we get to see how the characters navigate these conflicts.

I like to tie in Erik Erikson's psychosocial stages of development to the K-Drama characters we see because people can learn to better understand themselves when they see examples of it through

121

storytelling. I'm a clinician by training and I especially enjoy tying in psychological theory to get my point across. At the end of the day, my hope is to have people better understand themselves in relationship to their mental health, and to do that there are times I need to bring in my expertise. Erikson's theory points out that there's a crisis in each developmental stage experienced by the person in that season of life, but it's important to know that "crisis" here shouldn't be necessarily taken literally. It merely means the individual feels a conflict or some distress in that life stage and that conflict is misaligned with the life stage core value. Last year I did three Instagram reels on the psychosocial stages of development (see illustration) for folks to better understand what the "crisis" in each stage can look like.

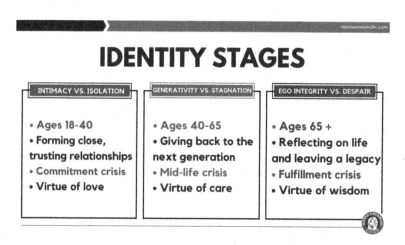

K-Dramas to Help You Understand a Midlife Crisis

That's the title of my first reel on identity stages, mainly because that's the stage that I and the majority of my clients and leaders that I coach are all part of. This reel was fairly popular, though it's important to note that this age group (40–65) isn't as active on social media and the platform they are most familiar with is Facebook. This being my age demographic, I understand this. In my flagship work on mental health and identity, I indicate that there is indeed such a thing as the midlife crisis since we are midlife age. This comment is generally met with a chuckle because what we tend to see in media is the trope of the "over-the-hill" folks doing something off the wall that's out of character. This age group is the "sandwich generation," raising kids and also looking after their aging parents. They're perhaps at a point in their lives where they are stopping to look at their career, family, and societal contributions and questioning why they're doing what they're doing or looking ahead to the future and wondering if they need to pivot. I see this in my work in both coaching and therapy.

K-Dramas showing good examples of this crisis:
- *Divorce Attorney Shin*
- *Our Blues*
- *18 Again*
- *A Gentleman's Dignity*
- *Second 20s*
- *On the Way to the Airport*
- *Second to Last Love*
- *When My Love Blooms*
- *Doctor Cha*
- *My Mister*

With more K-Drama fans around the world than ever before, the newer ones (2022–2023) tend to get the most feedback. I received a lot of messages on *Doctor Cha,* which I also enjoyed because I related personally to Doctor Cha. After more than 20 years of being a stay-at-home mother and wife to her doctor husband, Cha Jung Sook decides to go back to the workforce (she's in her late 40s or early 50s) and finish medical school residency. She had always wanted to be a doctor, but somewhere along the way she chose family over career. Her story is relatable in many ways since it wasn't just about pursuing a career, but about finding her own purpose and passion that makes her happy, and not living just for the sake of her children. Because it's typical in Asian culture to put the family first, particularly the children, Doctor Cha had a heartwarming take on her journey of self-discovery in her midlife crisis. As a family therapist, I really liked how the K-Drama shows us that we don't have to necessarily sacrifice either family or career to make things work. It can be a "both and." Hence, the dialectics. You can be 100% dedicated to your family but at the same time give 100% to your career. However, it's important to recognize that managing one's well-being is a priority. Doctor Cha shows us the conflict within and the guilt she felt (guilt is such a mainstay of Asian culture as well as of the working mom narrative) trying to be a successful resident in medical school. This conflict is important to see because she's grappling with the crisis in her identity stage but learning how to navigate it. Think back to the dialectics I described in an earlier chapter: you can experience polar opposite elements at the same time and that is okay.

There are times when a K-Drama hits too close to home for you to want to watch it. It's what I have heard from clients and followers, particularly over 2023's *Divorce Attorney Shin*. Several women I know had wanted to watch it because I was talking about at the time but worried it would be too painful because they had gone through divorce themselves. I pointed out that I liked how the show presents divorce particularly through the lens of a compassionate male divorce attorney who is on his own healing journey. So I recommend this particular K-Drama for its uplifting perspective on divorce.

Despite their hesitation, these viewers did end up enjoying this K-Drama. One of them ended up crying for days afterwards (which isn't necessarily what I want), but she had tried so hard to stay strong for the sake of her kids (who were in high school at the time) that she didn't realize how much she was holding in. Although the show did remind her of the pain of her divorce, she was finally able to move forward in her life, particularly when watching the scenes of Attorney Shin speaking to his clients. She related to different parts of the characters' stories, and it was her story that she was watching. And she saw how these characters were able to move on after divorce and find a new path of hope and happiness forward.

My favorite K-Drama is *My Mister*. I find the main character, Park Dong Hoon, inspirational. He is kind and generous, and he has integrity. When we meet him he is in a midlife crisis, unwittingly walking around discontent with his life and career. His indifference has driven a wedge between him and his wife, who ends up having an affair. But when 21-year-old Lee Jian enters his life, he finds a shift because he's able to focus on caring for her and giving back to the next generation. As I've mentioned, these are the values in this midlife stage, and when we first meet Dong Hoon, he is searching for that purpose. He's seeking the answer to a midlife question, "How can I contribute to society?" I'm highlighting this character because 1) he's an inspiring character for me, 2) he's an inspiring character for others to aspire to be, 3) we see his journey of growth and the confidence he gains by the end of the K-Drama, which is an example for folks in this midlife stage to learn from.

When people talk about *My Mister*, most refer to the female character of Jian, whose transformation is more obvious, but Dong Hoon is also transformed. The most difficult aspect of being stuck in a middle-age rut is regaining the spring in your step. Park Dong Hoon is able to do this despite finding out about his wife's affair. Yet despite it all, he is a great example of a team leader, and his reports respect him. Sometimes I point out how the characters in a particular K-Drama are examples of how we can choose to live our lives and how these characters navigate their challenges. In a sense through this "mentorship" of Jian, he discovered his worth. It enabled him to find a way to make a life-changing contribution and to define his own happiness. K-Dramas can show the most mundane of situations (which is why *My Mister* can be difficult for those who want a more active plot) and reveal the gold in a character's story that teaches us life lessons.

K-Dramas to Help You Understand an Older Adulthood Fulfillment Crisis

This reel focused on the aging population of the 65-plus age group. Because of the Asian cultural norms that respect and honor elders, K-Dramas do a beautiful job of showing their needs and crisis of fulfilment. Erikson's psychosocial stage for this demographic describes a value of wisdom and leaving a legacy. In the K-Dramas, we watch characters like the *halmuni* (grandma) and *harabugi* (grandpa) imparting wisdom to their younger family members while reflecting on their lives and what they have accomplished. The crisis of fulfillment asks, "Did I live a meaningful life? What do I have to show for it?"

K-Dramas showing examples of this crisis:
- *Dear My Friends*
- *My Father Is Strange*
- *Navillera*
- *My Unfamiliar Family*
- *Our Blues*
- *It's Beautiful Now*
- *Hometown Cha-Cha-Cha*
- *Once Again*
- *Reborn Rich*

A fan favorite from this list is *Dear My Friends,* where the main characters are of the aging population, which is rare to see. This show did a wonderful job of humanizing their experience. Although it was about the struggles surrounding the aging population, I have heard more about the response to this K-Drama from the young adult and middle-aged demographic. Young adults say they gained a better understanding of their parents' and grandparents' behaviors, especially when elders shared their opinions and were "stuck in their ways." They realize from this K-Drama that perhaps they felt valued and useful when imparting their life wisdom. Another poignant aspect of this K-Drama is the way the characters talk about aging and how they're having to wear adult diapers or losing loved ones and facing the realization that they're aging and can't do the things they were once able to. While we may know this of the aging demographic, to hear them sharing about it especially in the Asian culture is unique. We also see a storyline surrounding dementia and the difficulties for the caretaker, which can be meaningful to viewers who are dealing with this in their families. *Dear My Friends* shows us the perspective of the aging person with dementia, which isn't something we get to see often.

On my inaugural tour in September 2023, half of the participants were actually in this age demographic. They had a wealth of knowledge and also told me they love learning by watching K-Dramas. One 70-year-old participant stated, "K-Dramas keep my brain active, which I need at my age." She explained that she's constantly learning about the Korean culture and history when watching K-Dramas. Other folks around her age and older chimed in that if they want to know more about something they see in a K-Drama, they just google it. That's what keeps them current: they're eager not just to watch a K-Drama but also to glean something from it, especially when it relates to history. Another tour participant in the same age range indicated she loved the love story of 2021's *The Red Sleeve* so much that she had to do some digging to read about the tragic real-life story of King Jeongjo. Many folks also told me they enjoy historical K-Dramas and enjoy doing research to see whether the K-Drama has an accurate portrayal, and to understand the order of events, particularly during the Japanese colonization.

The underrated K-Drama *My Unfamiliar Family* presents a topic that is very important to the Korean culture. It's called *jolhon,* which basically means graduation from marriage, where married couples seek lives independent from each other without getting a divorce. The main reason is that it's easier to remain married for the sake of the family and finances. But also, especially among this age group, divorce has traditionally been taboo.

I was surprised when I heard the word *jolhon* in the first episode. The matriarch in this K-Drama is unhappy with her life and marriage and wants to graduate from marriage, much to the chagrin of her three adult children. This is an interesting angle from the aging demographic's perspective, especially since traditionally this age group got married fairly young and perhaps have never known what it's like to live on their own and be their own person. Clients and followers have told me how this K-Drama also helped them understand the marriage of their aging parents because they knew there was tension but didn't quite know the dynamics surrounding their parents' (or grandparents') relationship.

Other instructional K-Dramas in this vein are *Reborn Rich,* where the grandfather aggressively seeks to build a corporate conglomerate for the sake of his legacy, and *It's Beautiful Now,* where the grandfather creates a competition among his grandsons that whoever gets married first will get an apartment. This is also for the sake of expanding his family someday and having grandchildren, which is a big part of a family's legacy.

Finally, there's a scene in *Hometown Cha-Cha-Cha* that provides an example of how we can better understand the aging population, especially among the Asian community. This age group doesn't ask for help even when they need it desperately. They don't want to burden their children, so they hold in their pain, whether that's physical or emotional. I use the scene in episode three where Gamri, the beloved village halmuni, calls her son with the intention of asking for financial help to get tooth implants. She's been in pain for a while but hasn't done anything about it. Her son is given a heads-up by the male protagonist Chief Hong but doesn't give his mother a chance to ask for help, nor does he offer. She hears the busyness and impatience in his voice, and chooses not to speak up or mention her dental needs. It's a quick moment in the episode, but it's such a realistic example of our interactions with the aging population. Later on, her son regrets that he didn't spend more time with his mother, and I see this all too often.

K-Dramas to Help You Understand a Young Adult Crisis

This reel did the best when it came to views and going viral, but that's not surprising considering this demographic (ages 18–40) is most active on social media. The crisis in this life stage is about commitment, which echoes real life, as I see in my client's and follower's experiences. This is the age group where people consider finding a steady partner or life partner. This young adult stage asks, "Who can I love and who can love me?" As you can imagine, many K-Dramas resonate with this age group because love stories are central to K-Dramas. The most common questions I tend to get from clients and followers in this age group relate to relationships, from the idea of how realistic K-Drama relationships are, to whether it's okay to want to date a person like they see in K-Dramas, to comparing their own relationships to those in the shows, and also whether it's okay if they're in a relationship but have fluttering feelings for the K-Drama characters they watch. All these questions relate to their commitment crisis.

K-Dramas showing examples of this crisis:
- *Run On*
- *Weightlifting Fairy Kim Bok Joo*
- *Record of Youth*
- *Summer Strike*
- *When the Weather Is Fine*
- *Call It Love*
- *Hello, My Twenties*
- *Our Beloved Summer*
- *Twenty-Five Twenty-One*
- *My Mister*

- *Because This Is My First Life*
- *My Liberation Notes*
- *Start-Up*
- *Fight for My Way*

Each of these K-Dramas outlines a character's personal internal conflict, especially when it comes to being in a relationship with someone they care for or are in love with. The commitment crisis shows the character trying to navigate the struggle of loving someone and hoping they will be loved the same way in return. This life stage is about feeling isolated and alone and trying to find someone best suited for them, all the while trying to figure out who they are. In today's world, this is the Gen Z and Millennial population (or MZ Generation, as it's known in South Korea), who can most certainly identify with many K-Dramas because the themes center on committing to a relationship.

Twenty-Five Twenty-One was all the rage during the time of its airing but also for quite a bit of time afterwards, mainly because of the ending. In fact, I just met with a group of young professionals who brought up the ending and hashed it out again on what could've or should've happened. Without doing too much spoiling, let's say it's not an ending that this age group in particular wants to see, especially when they ask, "Will I be loved, or will I be alone?" The ending of this K-Drama is one I have talked about the most in the last year, because we don't necessarily get to see the main characters have that question answered. While there is a clear ending, we don't know how happy the characters are.

Though older age groups may have been hopeful for a usual K-Drama, they understood why *Twenty-Five Twenty-One* ended the way it did. However, the younger age groups seem to be troubled by the ending because the conflict of intimacy versus isolation isn't resolved. *Twenty-Five Twenty-One* really depicts the commitment crisis first-hand, which is a big deal to this age group and rightfully so.

For those between ages 18 and 40, their proficiency in social media spurred each other on over the ending because people continued to talk about it and commiserate. While I didn't want folks to stay upset, many in this age group tell me they're still bothered.

My Liberation Notes (another one of my personal favorites, written by the same writer as *My Mister*) resonates with many people, but particularly the MZ Generation in Korea because they find the everyday lives of the characters in this age group very relatable. Koreans related to *My Liberation Notes* in a different way than global viewers. They enjoyed seeing the portrayal of the siblings working, struggling with their long commute, living outside of Seoul because it's more affordable. All three live with their parents and feel the bane of their existence at times. In reality in Korea, this population struggles financially especially living in Seoul, where housing costs are so high. Koreans have told me they related to the characters' perspectives on their daily life and their relationships. Globally, the sentiment is similar except viewers related more to the relationship dynamics between the siblings, among the family, and the siblings' relationships with their love interests.

What put this drama on the map was a Korean word that created a lot of conversations about its exact meaning and what the writer intended. The female protagonist, Yeom Mi Jeong, tells the male protagonist, the famous Mr. Gu, that she wants him to *choo-ahng* her. The Netflix translation was "worship me," by which Mi Jeong is saying that love isn't enough. I spoke about its poignancy and how I preferred the word "cherish" rather than "worship," or in other translations, "reverence." I prefer "cherish" because this word reflects a behavior that is loving, rather than honoring. It's fascinating how that one word was the focal point of the drama, showing the perils and conflicts of young adulthood. Despite the K-Drama being very much about daily Korean life for that age group, globally people related to the emotions, the situations, and the behaviors of the characters.

Our Beloved Summer was another favorite, one I've used as an example of a realistic relationship that experiences growing pains. Both lead characters date in high school after doing a documentary together and their relationship continues on and off through college until the girl, Kook Yeon Soo, breaks up with Choi Woong. As anyone who's had high school relationships that didn't last after high school knows, this is a common scenario. What I particularly liked about this K-Drama was how, after their break-up, the main characters live their own lives, navigating their careers and learning about who they are, and then find themselves reunited, but in young adulthood this time. This question "Who can I love, and who can love me" is one that circles Yeon Soo and Choi Woong.

I use this K-Drama as an example of a healthy relationship, an answer to the burning question I get the most from this age group: "What are K-Drama examples of realistic relationships?" Theirs is one that especially embodies this, seeing their angst as they try to gauge each other's commitment. We're watching this crisis through-out the series until the time they're ready to take that step because they've matured. Finally, when Choi Woong heads to another country to expand his art portfolio while they're dating, that shows just how much the relationship has matured. They have both learned to place trust in their commitment to each other for the relationship to continue moving forward.

11

K-Dramas and Cultural Identity

Cultural identity refers to our belongingness to our culture—how we perceive our heritage, traditions, behavioral norms, language, and social practices. Because identity is always evolving, this is an ongoing process, involving how we internalize and connect with the core values, beliefs, and world schemas from our culture. In essence, our cultural identity is an important aspect of our self-concept, which directly correlates to our identity narrative. By now I'm sure you've gotten a strong sense that K-Dramas have made a tremendous impact on the Korean American and Asian American cultural identity and narrative, as well as on other cultural identity narratives.

I shared earlier how much the 1992 K-Drama *Jil-tu* (*Jealousy*) changed my life. In the 1980s and early 1990s, I knew very little about Korea and Korean culture and did not have a healthy perspective on my Korean American identity. *Jil-tu* was a foray into my culture, the first time I looked at my Korean American identity less critically, without so much disdain. I love when an Asian American "fan" who has seen me on social media enthusiastically speaks to me about how they love my take on K-Dramas for mental health because K-Dramas have given them a greater understanding of their cultural identity, which, in turn, helps their mental health.

One bubbly young lady on the subway in Seoul last year recognized me from TikTok and we had a terrific conversation. She talked excitedly about how she was born and raised in Toronto but did not feel connected to her Korean Canadian identity until recently, thanks to watching K-Dramas—a common narrative of many Korean Americans. The way K-Dramas have impacted her cultural identity is touching. Although she did grow up speaking Korean, it wasn't very good until she started watching more K-Dramas and practicing it more, and her growing proficiency in the language has helped tremendously in improving communication with her mother. As she started conversing with her mother more in Korean, her mother told her she feels like she can now tell her daughter everything she wanted to share with her while she was raising her but struggled to find the words due to the language barrier. This young lady is getting to know her mother better and learning more about her experience as an immigrant. She also told me how touched she was by an episode of *Hometown Cha-Cha-Cha* where Gamri (a village halmuni) calls her son to check in on him but he's too busy to have a conversation with her, as is her granddaughter. The young lady felt sad watching this, realizing she sometimes acts the same way with her own mother, and she called her up to check in on her. I felt so touched to hear this because it was yet another reminder of how K-Dramas bring an empathy and compassion to our relationships.

How does this connect to our cultural identity? She made such a mark on me during our brief subway conversation that it inspired me to write about her in my book because she was reconciling the cultural conflict between her Korean heritage and her Canadian upbringing. The joy in her face was evident as she was sharing with me how K-Dramas had given her a newfound appreciation for her Korean Canadian identity, as well as a greater peace in her relationship with her mother.

I'm part of some Korean American mommy groups on Facebook, where one of the most popular topics is discussing the K-Dramas they're watching with their families and which ones people recommend. I love seeing the discussion threads on Korean culture and the enthusiasm surrounding it. Although our community had been speaking about K-Dramas for decades, there's a different tone to our conversations in recent years. I can feel it and see it on the Facebook groups, and it makes me happy when mothers are discussing what their kids have gleaned from watching K-Dramas with them, or when they're planning a huge trip to Korea for the first time in years and they're just as excited as foreign tourists are. These groups are such an amazing place to talk about our culture and heritage through K-Dramas, and those outlets are very much needed as we shape and reshape our Korean American identity narrative.

A question I've been asked several times in interviews bothers me somewhat: "Did you decide to bring K-Dramas into your work with all the attention they've been getting?" The quick answer is no. By now you understand the meaning of K-Dramas in my life that made a smooth foray into my work. I brought K-Dramas into my sessions well before the pandemic and even talked about them with colleagues and fellow coaches, but wasn't taken seriously because no one outside the Asian community really knew about K-Dramas until 2020. There are so many implications in that question that I'm still trying to process it, and even as I write this I am full of emotion because there's still a misunderstanding. No, this was not about jumping on the bandwagon because of the popularity surrounding K-Dramas. I think because K-Dramas have made such an impact for me both personally and professionally, I get testy if someone assumes this was about being part of a trend. Cultural identity is a significant aspect of my flagship workshop on Cultural Confidence® to help people find the strength and confidence to defend and define their cultural identity when faced with questions like this.

A similar comment also makes me cringe inside (though I keep my smile bright): "I've noticed Korean Americans speaking up more about Korean culture and Korean content now that it's going global." Perhaps more people are noticing Korean Americans in relation to K-Culture and K-Content because they're more interested in K-Culture and K-Content. Korean Americans are not necessarily speaking up more, but they are being noticed more, so people are assuming they're speaking out more. When you ask someone questions or express interest in who they are, they'll be more apt to speak about their culture and heritage. Also, there's a rude implication that Korean Americans or even Asian Americans are somehow taking advantage of the global popularity of K-Dramas, K-Pop, and K-Beauty. I also assume from this comment that we wouldn't even get noticed if it hadn't been for K-Culture accomplishments. This is why I say that the K-Content phenomenon is a double-edged sword.

Perhaps it looks like Korean Americans are popping up all over the place because people are looking for anything related to Korean culture and South Korea because they're interested in it.

Cultural identity and the belongingness we have to our own culture is a complicated subject. Our identity narrative includes the internal cultural conflict we experienced growing up. I speak and educate passionately on the intersectionality of mental health and identity because it's what grounds us in our inner being. To be successful leaders in our fields, we need to take pride in our cultural identity even as it's evolving. Much of the immigrant experience has to do with feeling like a perpetual foreigner in one's own host country. We will continue experiencing challenges in our cultural identity and our relationship thereof, which is why it's important to know we are experts about ourselves. We can define our narrative in a way that works for us.

Filial Piety

Much of the family angst in K-Dramas stems from the stressors of filial piety (*hyo* or *hyodo* in Korean), which is a profound element of our identity and its link to our mental health, particularly in Asian culture. Filial piety is a central virtue of Confucianism, the values of which, as I explained in an earlier chapter, are at the core of Korean society. Other core tenets of Confucianism are also evident in K-Dramas, including an emphasis on education, self-development, peace and harmony, and loyalty. Though it has Asian roots, filial piety is a universal concept, and people of various ethnicities feel its pressures, which is why I believe it resonates when they see it in K-Dramas.

Filial piety is the deep-rooted sense of obligation we feel to serving and pleasing our parents, families, elders, and ancestors. It's about bringing respect and honor to the family, and at its core it's about intergenerationality. The pressure to prioritize your family, particularly having to follow your parents' wishes for you, is indeed a stressor felt in many families, as we see in K-Dramas. When they feel like they're a disappointment to their parents and elders, as we see in K-Dramas, there's a lot of shame and guilt. Filial piety resonates for many people, and much of my own behavior and decision-making stemmed from filial piety.

Squid Game, 2021

There are many examples of filial piety in K-Dramas, some more obvious than others. One small but powerful example appears in the famous 2021 *Squid Game.* In the second episode, we see Cho Sang Woo, the childhood friend of the male protagonist Seong Gi Hun, hiding while watching his mother work at her market booth from afar. He's checking up on her but cannot face her because he's ashamed of the large debt he's accrued. Gi Hun's words in the next scene highlight the pressures he feels. He tells Sang Woo that he should just tell his mother about his debt knowing he can regain the money by continuing to work. Even though he's a grown adult, the deep-rooted sense of duty to please his mother and honor her for raising him with his work and money propels him to attempt suicide, and then later to participate in the *Squid Game,* all to earn back the money he lost so he doesn't have to disappoint his mother, who's so proud of him.

When I discuss his story in my workshops, I explain that Sang Woo makes deadly choices throughout the K-Drama because of the shame and guilt surrounding what he thinks is a major failure in his life (falling into debt) and failing to make his mother proud. This is all assumed, since she has no idea of any of this. In the meantime, to emphasize my point about the gravity of distress that filial piety can bring, I mention that we see her telling everyone proudly that her son is doing great things in the United States working in finance, so we can only imagine that when he hears this when he's around her, it would add to the stress not to disappoint. Parental boasting is also an aspect of filial piety that only perpetuates the distress for the child, whether young or old.

It's a pattern we see in many families, particularly Asian. As small as this example of filial piety is (one or two scenes), Sang Woo shows he will stop at nothing to win the cash prize, all so he can bring that cash back to his mother and be the dutiful son she expects him to be. Sang Woo's desperation reflects real life. In Korea, the strong sense of duty to honor one's family has a direct relationship to the high number of suicides. Korea has the highest suicide rate among the OECD—people would rather die than bring shame to the family.

This example of filial piety has become a mainstay in flagship workshops. It's a subtle but powerful way to make my point. Following one of my workshops on K-Drama and mental health, a gentleman in his early 40s told me he relates to Sang Woo. He hadn't watched *Squid Game* but had heard of it and was eager to watch it after I described it in the workshop. He was at a breaking point because he was miserable in his career as a corporate attorney, but he kept at it because he was supporting his parents and his younger sister, who has Down syndrome. He was the first one in his extended family to attend college (an Ivy League university at that) and knew how proud his parents were that he became a lawyer and did all the right things, until he felt so lonely and isolated. Because he dedicated everything to his parents and extended family and to his busy career, he didn't have time for a relationship, which he desire. He declared to me that he felt like he was on Sang Woo's path and didn't want to end up like him. (I had described in my workshop how Sang Woo ends up, indicating a spoiler alert.) It's always hard for me when folks share their stories with me on the spot after my workshops. But besides listening and validating, what I was able to do for him was refer him to a therapist in his local area, and recommend he seek counseling to help him navigate the pressures he felt to make the best decisions for himself. He was not Asian, but he completely related to the concept of filial piety and told me he appreciated that he now has a term for what he had felt all these years. He left feeling hopeful and armed with a slew of other K-Dramas to watch for mental health.

Crash Course in Romance, 2023

This is another wonderful K-Drama that shows the stressors and extreme pressures of the education system in Korea. It also offers a great example of filial piety that many of my clients and followers pointed out because they struggled with a mother's behavior toward her second son. We see a driven mother who's an attorney and estranged from her husband, which we assume has a lot to do with her behavior and parenting their boys. The second son is a dutiful one. He follows what his mother says he should do and is a top student in his school—the perfect son, or *hyoja* as we say in Korean. But he's struggling with all the pressure, especially because his older brother is a school dropout. We see his mother double up on pressure, attention, and demand on the younger son.

While many viewers empathized with the son, it should be remembered that filial piety is a thread throughout all generations, so the mother most likely also experienced it from her parents and is transferring it to her son. So it's an interesting example of filial piety to watch the mother change her ways (as K-Dramas show so well in character development) for the sake of her son, who confronts her after he buckles from all the stress over getting into college.

The biggest conflict I see in families is a parent's desire for a child's future career and family that differs from that of their children. Many of my clients are bitter and angry because of the stressors surrounding filial piety. My role is to help them through this bitterness and anger and hope there's a way to heal the family relationship for the sake of everyone's mental health. This is what we see happen in *Crash Course in Romance*. It's not the main storyline, but it's a profound one and the poignancy of it left many viewers enjoying the mother-son dynamic. They took away a lesson for their own lives on how to be an authoritative parent (nurturing and firm), not an authoritarian one (my way or the highway). From the child's perspective, followers have told me they aspired to be like the son and make decisions that work for them, all the while communicating with their parents about it.

Boys Over Flowers, 2009

A gateway K-Drama for many, *Boys Over Flowers* presents us with an obvious depiction of filial piety. Viewers greatly dislike the mother, who schemes and plots throughout the drama in order to ensure her son, Gu Jun Pyo, takes over the company conglomerate and marries into a family that matches their social and financial status. Their relationship is strained (no surprise) and things are more complicated when he falls in love with Geum Jandi, whose parents own a dry cleaner, and she is on a swim scholarship in order to attend his school. Although it's not obvious, much of the K-Drama's plot centers on the mother-son conflict. He tries to be a dutiful son (hyoja), doing his best to honor his family and business, while trying to fight for what he wants, which is to be with the person he loves.

The mother's behavior is interesting because she's so focused on what she believes is best for the family and especially for her son that she doesn't really know him. This is what Jandi points out to his mother when he lands in the hospital after an accident. I talk about filial piety via *Boys Over Flowers* to show parents how jarring it can look—parents often do not know how their behavior comes across because they're so focused on protecting the family that it can blind them to hearing from their children about what they actually need. Sometimes parents take what I say literally and think that I mean they're supposed to approve every relationship just because it's what their children want or give in to all their children's wishes. So I explain that I'm pointing out filial piety in *Boys Over Flowers* or other K-Dramas as a way to show examples of how this concept manifests in a family and what it does to strain the relationship and create discord and distance, which is the last thing parents and children want. Parents should definitely share their opinions about their children's career and family choices, but should also recognize that it can be a process of mutuality and not a top-down approach to change family patterns that do not work. It's important for parents to remember the pressures they themselves were faced with as children so they can engage with their own children in what could be challenging conversations.

K-Dramas That Show What Filial Piety Looks Like:
- *Sky Castle*
- *Boys Over Flowers*
- *Crash Course in Romance*
- *Squid Game*
- *Something in the Rain*
- *True Beauty*
- *Itaewon Class*
- *Young Lady and Gentleman*
- *One Spring Night*
- *Crash Landing on You*
- *The Red Sleeve*
- *Reply 1988*

Acculturation

Acculturation is the process of adjusting and adapting to the prevailing or dominant culture. It directly impacts one's emotional, social, and psychological well-being when seeking to assimilate to the host culture in which they reside. I hear from many immigrants, both clients and followers, about how K-Dramas have helped them reflect on their acculturation experience, and that of their parents. That's not the word they use, but it's the term for what they're describing to me.

As I've discussed before, the global appeal of K-Dramas lies within the themes and messages surrounding culture, identity, resilience, trauma, healing, and hope, which describes the immigrant experience. This is the experience of my parents, and the cultural change surrounding their acculturation of course impacted me. We don't necessarily see examples of acculturation in K-Dramas since it's a homogenous culture. Yet the concept resonates for many specifically due to watching K-Dramas, because seeing the emotions that arise in the characters from their experiences evokes the viewers' own emotions, social interactions, and psychological impact surrounding our acculturation narrative. What we're watching and how we process it—in areas such as behavior, nonverbal and verbal communication, social interactions, and cultural nuances—speaks to us. K-Content *Forbes* writer Joan MacDonald says she's learned a lot about "what it was like to be an American" from watching K-Dramas since she's an immigrant herself, having emigrated from the Netherlands when she was six years old. She says, "Television is a very powerful medium that helps you understand things about a culture, even if it's not realistic."

The content creator @maxnotbeer shares how much he enjoyed both seasons of *Hospital Playlist,* crying his way through it. He resonates with it because he considered himself "an extremely dependent person" and didn't imagine a life on his own as he's doing now. He says that watching the doctor best friends going through life's up and downs and getting through it together has helped him do what he's doing today, making a living in Korea as a Jewish American content creator. Max also spoke about how he loves *Reply 1988,* which "strikes such a deep chord" because it's all about the family, which directly ties into his Jewish identity, of which he is proud.

Max speaks highly of his Jewish heritage. Its strong similarities to Korean culture make him feel comfortable as a content creator covering Korean culture, and it's why he feels it's natural to be living in Korea. What he's speaking about is his own acculturation experience. Max's adjustment to living in Korea was smooth because of the belongingness he feels to the Korean culture and its strong ties to his Jewish culture. Max explains that a core tenant of Judaism is hospitality, which he also sees as a core tenant in Korean culture. This is what we also see in our K-Dramas. He finds that both cultures lean into hospitality, welcoming guests with food and warmth, and with "open arms."

Max told me he had no trouble living with a host family back in 2017 because they acted like his own family would, regardless of language barrier. A common theme we see in K-Dramas is how the characters overcome barriers and obstacles in the acculturation process to achieve their successes, which Max says is the tie-in between Jewish and Korean history. He finds that both of our histories have strong commonalities, including facing prejudice and discrimination, and being targeted by neighbors. He shares, "The Seoul I live in now and fell in love with was basically built from ruins, from the ground up." He says that because he's Jewish, he resonates very deeply with the idea that despite the tragedy and hardships Korea faced, its history, culture, and traditions have thrived under the toughest of conditions." His story brought tears to my eyes because I could see first-hand what an emotional investment he has in Korea, again because he relates so profoundly as a Jewish American.

Max's story is similar to what I hear from many other folks of different ethnicities who relate to K-Drama stories and tie it back to their acculturation experience. A Nigerian mother told me she learns so much from K-Dramas, specifically *Mr. Sunshine* (one of my top favorite K-Dramas of all time) in understanding more about her immigrant experience. She related to Mr. Sunshine's (Eugene Choi) disdain for Korea, and the fact that he felt betrayed because his own country didn't take care of him. She couldn't quite pinpoint exactly why she related to this. I told her she doesn't have to understand the why per se, but she should recognize that there's some resentment in her acculturation experience, which is still unfolding. When someone leaves their country of origin and moves to another country, they're focused on surviving (before thriving), learning a new language, understanding the nuances of a new culture and its people. There's so much to this experience and the complexity runs deep. Watching a K-Drama storyline can perhaps unveil what's underneath you in layers like an onion, peeling one by one while crying until you figure out what is at the core.

Mr. Sunshine, 2018

Mr. Sunshine is a staple K-Drama in my identity workshops. Eugene Choi, the male protagonist, is an officer in the U.S. Army in the early 1900s. He fled South Korea with an American missionary when he was a little boy after his parents were murdered by their rich land-owner employers. Those same employers hire folks to hunt him down, so Eugene has understandably been left scarred and we see this in his narrative. Eugene comes back to Korea during the Japanese colonization, proudly representing the United States. His journey is beautiful as he falls in love with a Korean noblewoman who is passionately fighting for the freedom of Joseon (Korea) and he doesn't understand why. Through her passion for and dedication to Korea, he comes to learn about the country he came from and finds healing in his own acculturation and identity journey. This is an absolutely brilliant K-Drama that I highly recommend. It's an excellent representation of the emotions surrounding acculturation and the conflict one has with a country they left and no longer recognize. Although it's a Korean drama, *Mr. Sunshine* showcases the immigrant experience in all its poignancy and poeticism. I won't spoil the ending to this one, but he comes to a reconciliation of sorts that brings an inner healing, which impacts the decisions he makes in the end. I'm getting chills sharing about this story. I have heard from many people who are non-Korean, even non-Asian, that they resonate with *Mr. Sunshine* because they see their parents or themselves in Eugene Choi.

Adoptee Narratives

My work with K-Dramas has brought me closer to the Asian adoptee community, especially Korean adoptees. I met many adoptees during the pandemic, especially on the audio app Clubhouse, where I hosted talks on K-Dramas for mental health. I have found their stories so touching, but sad, especially when I hear them talking wistfully about K-Dramas that they're so happy to have discovered. But they're sad at the same time because they're learning wonderful things about a culture and country they hadn't really known. I have often heard they wished they could have learned about Korea sooner, or started watching K-Dramas sooner, to soak up all they can about their heritage. I've told some folks that it's never too late because they can catch up now in the present moment. But understandably it's still hard for them to accept.

One Korean adoptee told me *Crash Landing on You* was her foray into Korean culture, and she couldn't believe all these years she had been disinterested in her heritage until she watched that K-Drama. She hadn't realized how significant representation was for her until that moment. She hasn't looked back, and only eagerly looked forward to learning all that she can to catch up on what she had missed about Korean culture. Another adoptee told me she feels like an emotional dam burst when she started watching K-Dramas and emotions just pour out each time she watches one and learns something else about Korea and Korean culture. She never knew she had a connection but feels one while watching K-Dramas. Suddenly, she's ravenous for all things Korean. She has been lucky to visit several times in the last few years and hopes to live in Korea someday. Another adoptee told me he started watching K-Dramas after hearing me talk about them on Clubhouse. He has a good relationship with his adoptee parents, but found that he struggles because they chose not to share about his Korean culture or expose to him to any experiences surrounding his heritage.

I met one Asian adoptee at the start of the pandemic who had begun leaning more into her adoptee narrative thanks to meeting more fellow adoptees on the Clubhouse app. She and I got friendly since she had been watching K-Dramas for some time. Based on our conversations, I suggested she rewatch the 2014 K-Drama *Healer,* which features an adoptee storyline that I thought was well done, but I wanted her opinion as an adoptee. She was excited about this assignment because she felt that her relationship to her adoptee identity had shifted in recent years and believed she would see the K-Drama in a different light. *Healer* was one of her favorite K-Dramas, so she was curious to see her reaction watching it at this time. Sure enough, a couple of weeks later she told me while she still enjoyed the K-Drama overall, she cringed at some moments surrounding the main character's current narrative with her beloved adopted father. She hadn't noticed it when she first watched but felt that the K-Drama fantasized a bit in how loving her adopted father was and how happy a life she has with her adopted father. Also, she felt that the character's "reunion" with her birth mother was too simplified and downplayed the complexities of the adoptee narrative because they may be conflicted and unsure about how they feel toward their birth parents. Basically, she found that she felt differently about the K-Drama than she initially had felt because of where she was in her own adoptee identity journey.

I have also told Korean adoptees that Korean Americans who have been exposed to the culture all their lives have similar regrets. In my line of work, I have found a similarity in the Korean adoptee experience and the Korean American experience when it comes to their cultural identity. Both have kept a distance, the latter choosing to do so due to cultural conflict and assimilation, either pushed by their parents or desired by themselves. Adoptees weren't really given a choice; hence their eagerness, sometimes even desperation, to grasp at all things Korean culture saddens me. They're making up for lost time, as they tell me. Without assuming I know what it's like to be an adoptee, I relate in some ways because I also am making up for lost time since I had chosen to disengage from Korean culture until young adulthood. A few Korean adoptees told me they cried when they visited Korea for the first time since they had been adopted as a baby. They also cried several times throughout their trip visiting their birthplace, participating in Korean activities, and enjoying the food. They felt a connection, a "chemical reaction" they experienced being in Korea, like visiting an old friend they hadn't seen in a very long time but had known for years.

This makes sense. I defined identity at the beginning of this chapter as a psychological attachment. It gives us belongingness, meaning, and purpose, so regardless of what people may think or feel about their cultural heritage, it's something we desire to connect to regardless of our upbringing, background, and exposure to it.

K-Dramas Showing Adoptee Narratives:

- *Vincenzo*
- *Healer*
- *Thirty-Nine*
- *Her Private Life*
- *I'm Sorry, I Love You*
- *Mr. Sunshine*
- *Kill Me, Heal Me*
- *Doctor Cha*
- *Pinocchio*
- *Move to Heaven (ep. 9)*
- *When the Weather Is Fine*
- *Our Beloved Summer*

12

K-Dramas and Neurodiversity

We are all neurodivergent. That's according to Ellie Middleton, who's known as an expert on supporting disabled communities. She also runs the unmasked community for neurodivergence. Middleton indicates that there are neurotypical people whose functioning falls within societal norms and standards, and neurodivergent people are those whose functioning falls outside of those norms, including those on the autism spectrum, and those with ADHD and dyslexia. Several prominent K-Dramas feature neurodivergent people, specifically those on the autism spectrum, such as *Crash Course in Romance*, *Extraordinary Attorney Woo*, *Move to Heaven*, *It's Okay to Not Be Okay*, and *The Good Doctor*.

Extraordinary Attorney Woo, 2022

This K-Drama gained mass attention in South Korea as well as around the world. It was the feel-good show that everyone needed at the time as the pandemic was turning into an endemic. As one of the K-Dramas in recent years that has made a positive impact on Korean society, *Attorney Woo* brought more awareness to neurodiversity, which historically hasn't been addressed properly in Korea. It was met with some criticism from the autistic community for what they felt was a somewhat unrealistic portrayal because the female protagonist Woo Young Woo is on the high end of the autism spectrum, but overall her portrayal was well received. I believe *Attorney Woo* did so well because the character was aspiring, she was adorably cute, and she was trying to find her way in the world as a new attorney. She worked hard to get there and faced obstacles along the way as she defended her clients in the best way she knew how.

Extraordinary Attorney Woo promoted many conversations surrounding neurodiversity and disability awareness, and a greater understanding of what it looks like and how to support it. The supportive team environment in this K-Drama embodied positivity in the workplace and everyone being given a fair chance to succeed—it's always good for our mental health to see this. The acronym DEIB comes to mind: diversity, equity, inclusion, belonging. I am a DEIB consultant in the workplace and I believe this K-Drama's Hanbada Law Firm is a workplace to emulate. Her boss displays realistic skepticism, and the colleague who dislikes her, thinking she has an unfair advantage and gets things the easy way, also displays a realistic attitude of what we may experience in the workplace.

In the end, Woo Young Woo manages to use her skills, strengths, and sense to do her best for her clients. As portrayed in the K-Drama, she is the first lawyer who has autism in South Korea (perhaps in all of Asia) who happened to graduate from the top law school in the country and her genius shows. While she may have the smarts to match any top colleague in her field, Young Woo shows us her struggles, both social and emotional, that come with her autism. I have many lawyer friends who are K-Drama fans and enjoyed watching *Attorney Woo*. While they were sometimes skeptical of the legal semantics happening in the courtroom scenes, overall they thought it was a great K-Drama. The many stories meshed into the overarching story of this show also make it a fan favorite. We were rooting for Young Woo to win cases (she doesn't win them all) and to see her be given a fair chance in the courtroom.

I have added *Extraordinary Attorney Woo* to my list of K-Dramas that I use in my corporate workshops, particularly showing Young Woo claiming her neurodivergent status as a person with autism. This is how the K-Drama kicks off, which I think is brilliant, and as a therapist, I would have wanted Young Woo to handle it the way she did. She faces stigma in the very difficult environment of the courtroom, indicating she is a person with autism. This forestalls the uncomfortable questioning she could have received surrounding her behavior in social situations and stating what could have been obvious, which shows courageousness and confidence. The stigma surrounding mental health and mental illness tends to come from avoidance or lack of understanding because it isn't explained. Woo Young Woo takes that away, which gave others the ability to focus on *her* ability.

I especially enjoyed reading an interview in The *Korea Herald* with Haley Moss, who deeply resonated with Young Woo because she happens to be Florida's first practicing lawyer with autism, and she appreciated Young Woo talking openly about autism from the onset. Moss particularly related to how Young Woo's colleagues first treated her, which is similar to what Moss experienced in the workplace as she was first starting out. She also appreciated seeing Young Woo's autistic traits, such as wearing headphones because she's sensitive to noise, and eating kimbap every day. Moss says she also wears headphones because she gets anxious around loud noises, and she eats a lot of the same foods each day as well. Moss also has a "near-photographic" memory like Young Woo does and the "exceptional ability" to connect people and places that give her the edge as a lawyer. What Moss most appreciated was seeing Young Woo in a mainstream setting, learning and growing with the other lawyers; rather than being alone in a separate place, she is part of the Hanbada Law Firm and a valued lawyer at that. Moss was glad to see a K-Drama like *Attorney Woo*, and hopeful that there'll be more like it.

One of my dedicated followers whom I have gotten to know over the last year was diagnosed with autism a couple of years ago, right around the time *Attorney Woo* was airing. This surprised me because of her age, which is older than the norm, but she tells me the diagnosis is better late than never. She felt relieved when she was diagnosed, because everything finally made sense to her when it came to her behavior and thinking, and what she questioned about herself. She also appreciated *Extraordinary Attorney Woo*, which, because of her new diagnosis, was a timely K-Drama that she found very validating and boosted her confidence even more when it came to her diagnosis. This is a reminder of how powerful representation is; seeing a replica of yourself on screen helps you feel seen and heard, which is what we all desire.

Remember my gal pal Hiromi Okuyama? She's the one who turned to K-Dramas during a distressing time in her life because she felt bad for bothering me. Hiromi's second K-Drama happened to be *Extraordinary Attorney Woo* because many of her American friends recommended it to her. Hiromi didn't want to watch it at first because she has a son who's on the spectrum, and in her words she's seen "so many" videos on autism. However, she decided to watch it and it brought her to tears, but also brought many chuckles and laughs because she saw her own son in Woo Young Woo. She appreciated Young Woo's "cute quirks," and the "sweet" interactions in her relationships was an angle Hiromi hadn't seen in all the videos she's watched. It was the first time she could laugh about anything related to autism and it felt refreshing to laugh because everything was relatable. She was able to recall fondly some of her son's behaviors that she had fretted over, and seeing it from Woo Young Woo comforted her.

Hiromi felt *Extraordinary Attorney Woo* humanized those on the spectrum and normalized the behavior that people tend to struggle with. For instance, she loved seeing Young Woo's obsession with kimbap to show how the brain functions for neurodivergent people. Her son is the same way, and it made her feel more of a fondness toward her son instead of seeing his behaviors as an inconvenience or embarrassment. Watching this K-Drama also helped her realize that perhaps she herself could be on the spectrum because she felt like there was "something always weird about her" when she was little. She didn't just relate to Young Woo from the perspective of a mother of a child with autism but found the behavior like that of her own.

Extraordinary Attorney Woo has that effect on many like it did on Hiromi. In my experience, it's the first one in the history of K-Dramas to have a fully global effect, where it was top rated not only in South Korea but around the world. Generally, the trend has been that when a K-Drama is popular in the United States or other Western countries, it doesn't resonate on the same level in South Korea, and vice versa. This K-Drama brought an awareness among Korean society like never before because of its memorable and iconic portrayal of a main character who's neurodivergent. And globally, it spurred on more conversations surrounding neurodivergence and ableism, which can make for heated discussions, but for DEIB in the workforce, community, and schools, these conversations are necessary for impactful change.

The Powerful Intersectionality of K-Dramas and Resilience

13 | K-Dramas and the Workplace

A young lady on my inaugural tour last year—let's call her Rachael—told me she was a different person on my tour. She had not felt that relaxed for as long as she could recall. For instance, she dropped her phone at one of the tour sites and cracked it. Normally, this would have stressed her out, but she wasn't fazed by it, telling herself it wasn't a big deal. This reaction surprised her at the time since that hadn't been the nature of her behavior to that point. Rachael explained that leading up to the tour she had been struggling at her work and extremely burned out, disillusioned, and close to quitting until she heard about my tour and jumped at the chance. I would like to say I was the reason for her happier, calmer, and more peaceful mood. But I told her I believed it had to do with the fact that she got to take a break by being with like-minded people on vacation, all there for the same reason: K-Drama fans eager to visit South Korea for the first time. She got to be across the ocean on another continent and leave her work behind for a much-needed respite. Rachael was surrounded by a safe community, not isolated nor alone.

What I was most happy to hear about was how her mindset shifted during the tour. She was grounded in each moment, enjoying the present instead of dreading having to go back to work, which is something she had expected to feel when a vacation ends. Instead, she found herself taking it day by day, soaking in the fun as she made new friends around her age, and came back to work refreshed and rejuvenated. We both knew it didn't necessarily mean her workplace would be the best fit for her in the time to come, but it meant she got to prioritize her mental health and fully enjoy herself, all the while being in the company of fellow K-Drama fans. I was so moved by her tour experience because one of the core aspects of my work is being a corporate speaker on workplace mental health. I advocate for trips such as this, especially when people work from home, for the sake of workplace well-being. Rachael needed to be in a warm environment in the company of people who related to her regardless of stage of life. I am so thankful she found it on my tour.

That said, I knew I had hit the next level in my work with using K-Dramas for mental health when I was contacted by two women who worked in the legal department at a huge corporation headquartered in St. Petersburg, Florida. They had been following me on social media, and fresh off the *Extraordinary Attorney Woo* faze, they wanted to bring me in to speak on mental health for the legal team, using *Attorney Woo* as well as any other K-Dramas that I wanted to include in my workshop. This was very special to me for many reasons. Up until that point, I was speaking on K-Dramas for mental health at events and conferences mainly for Asian Pacific Islander audiences. Yet here I was being contacted by the legal team at a global corporation for a non-Asian audience of attorneys and paralegals, including the chief counsel of the organization. It was such a privilege and honor working with these lovely ladies, so I was already enjoying the pre-event experience. Being there in St. Petersburg in October 2022 was a highlight of my clinical career to date. I was thrilled to be speaking about K-Dramas for mental health in front of an audience where that topic might be unexpected. A small group of people had been watching K-Dramas when I polled the audience, but as we know, when K-Drama fans get together, they tend to win over their colleagues slowly but surely. I appreciated seeing the enthusiasm over K-Dramas and acknowledging the connection to mental health. Facing a straitlaced corporate work environment can be challenging, but using K-Dramas as an icebreaker to warm up the crowd has proven to be working. It goes back to the very reason why Noona's Noonchi came about in the first place: to use K-Dramas to promote more conversations around mental health for the sake of normalizing and destigmatizing it.

Another highlight was presenting a similar workshop for H&M, which wanted me to show K-Dramas for mental health and highlight AAPI mental health and identity for the month of May. This is my busiest month since it's National Mental Health Awareness month as well as AANHPI Heritage Month in the United States. I presented my flagship workshop on mental health and Asian identity using K-Drama examples throughout. Many in my audience had not heard of K-Dramas, but that didn't matter because I'm not there to promote watching K-Dramas; I'm using K-Dramas as a tool to understand and address mental health and mental illness, as well as to normalize conversations on the subject. The most fun part of my workshops is the preparation, when I spend time finding the right K-Drama examples (clips of scenes) to illustrate my points. It's enjoyable for obvious reasons, but also allows me the boost I need for my own mental health, since that's why I watch K-Dramas in the first place.

"We Decided to Create a K-Drama Club at Work!"

I am hearing more and more about K-Drama groups in the workplace. Even though I talk about K-Dramas for mental health, this still boggles my mind, and I'm so happy to hear it and to take part in helping to change the landscape in the workforce if I'm able to. Much of my work in DEIB is with employee resource groups (ERGs), also known as business resource groups (BRGs) or affinity groups. I believe they play an important role in workplace well-being. They enhance corporate culture and provide belongingness in the workplace, which builds trust and fosters employee engagement. From what I am seeing and hearing, K-Drama clubs are the same way. A follower said she decided to start a K-Drama club at work after watching *My Liberation Notes,* in which the female protagonist struggles with being part of an after work "club" because she doesn't relate to any of the available ones, so she decides to start her own with two other colleague who weren't part of clubs either. This sparked my follower's interest to do the same at her work, even if it started with just three of them. I asked her if it has enhanced her work experience, to which she replied, "You bet it does! We love coordinating our in-office workdays so we can talk about K-Dramas in person. Plus, our coworkers end up stopping by to see what we're having so much fun laughing about!" Yes, I am endorsing the idea of starting a K-Drama club at work. Perhaps it can be another ERG (or BRG), since those groups can also be designed to bring folks together with similar hobbies and interests.

Remember, I am not promoting K-Drama itself; I am promoting K-Dramas for mental health, especially in the workplace, which is what I speak about the most as a corporate speaker.

According to Mind Share Partners' latest (2021) report on mental health at work, burnout, depression, and anxiety have increased by 40%, with burnout increase being the highest at 56%. Interestingly, burnout wasn't part of their previous workplace mental health report. This data aligns with what I have been seeing the past few years, but I believe the numbers are even higher and we will most likely see that reflected in future data (as of this writing the 2023 data hasn't been released yet). It's assumed that the most difficult time was during the pandemic itself. But I tell organizations and their executives that it's post-pandemic, and that's challenging because of what we all went through during the pandemic. I am seeing the ripple effects of the global pandemic now more than ever. What I find fascinating, but not surprising, is seeing how K-Dramas have come into the fold in all sectors of the workplace as a form of self-care and team building. And I include that in my own data because it contributes to the bottom line, as I tell leaders and professionals.

My work isn't just in corporate, but also very much in the nonprofit sector, universities, and communities. Being a clinician, I have been collecting my own qualitative data as I enter these workplaces, both in person and virtually, to provide education on workplace mental health. In the last couple of years, I have brought in K-Dramas for mental health in nearly 70% of my workshops and sessions.

Here's a summary of what I have been discussing throughout this book: how K-Dramas can promote happier and healthier workplaces for successful business outcomes:

- **Mindfulness practice:** K-Dramas' stories and characters make for light-hearted conversations at work, offering positive distractions for professionals and leaders, and grounding them in the present moment for a healthier mindset toward their jobs.

- **Psychological safety:** K-Dramas enhance camaraderie and build rapport among colleagues and leaders, which leads to greater trust and accountability.
- **Managing stress to prevent burnout:** K-Dramas (a dose a day) are a great form of self-care and coping mechanism to manage daily stress levels so burnout doesn't happen.
- **Leadership and professional development:** K-Drama stories and their depth of character development provide terrific examples of workplace best practices and workplace leadership.
- **Mental health awareness:** K-Dramas help normalize conversations surrounding mental health and educate on mental illness (they're not the same). K-Dramas are a unique way of talking about difficult issues, while not making it about yourself since you're referring to the characters in the shows.
- **Belongingness at work:** K-Dramas provide a welcoming space for shared experiences to promote DEIB because everyone can find commonalities in the stories and characters, as well as tie them back to the workplace. This especially includes marginalized communities, such as people of color and the queer community.

K-Dramas Showing Queer Characters and Storylines:
- *Love in Contract*
- *Itaewon Class*
- *Run On*
- *Hometown Cha-Cha-Cha*
- *Mine*
- *Dinner Mate*
- *Be Melodramatic*
- *Coffee Prince*

Although my work is still met with some skepticism at times, for the most part I generally feel supported and even encouraged by those who hear about what I do. Several years ago it wasn't this way.

I did not share with organizations that I brought K-Dramas into my sessions or use them as mental health deep dives, because, as I've indicated throughout this book, until recently K-Dramas were known only to a select group of communities and people weren't necessarily ready to learn more about them until the pandemic hit. As the demand grows for my speaking on K-Dramas for mental health, my confidence has grown too. This is where I like to say that practice makes progress. Because I curate all my content, customizing my workshops based on the audience I am presenting to, I have a lot of data and research up my sleeve to be able to win audiences over. Again, my ultimate goal is not to promote K-Dramas for their own sake, but to promote them as a tool to benefit your mental health, an effective coping mechanism for daily mental health hygiene. There's a K-Drama for everyone and, as I like to joke, "The only drama in your life should be a K-Drama."

K-Dramas That Show Healthy Workplace Relationships:
- *Extraordinary Attorney Woo*
- *Business Proposal*
- *My Mister*
- *Call It Love*
- *Search: WWW*
- *Descendants of the Son*
- *Vincenzo*
- *Jinny's Kitchen* (reality show)
- *Romance Is a Bonus Book*
- *Divorce Attorney Shin*
- *Itaewon Class*
- *Taxi Driver*
- *Start-Up*
- *Tomorrow*
- *Hospital Playlist*
- *Coffee Prince*

14 | K-Dramas = Belongingness + Jeong

What makes K-Dramas unique? I've heard this question repeatedly and my answer has remained the same. It's Jeong, as you heard me discuss earlier in the book, and I cannot think of a better way to conclude than by talking about the experience of Jeong, which is a core tenet in the K-Drama experience that benefits our mental health. Jeong refers to the poignant emotional sentiment of love, connection, belongingness, fondness, kinship, and more. Jeong is innate in Korean society, something you can see in K-Dramas, but also something you very much feel.

There are powerful and conflicting emotions surrounding Jeong. Although it can be an uplifting, encouraging sentiment, there are times it can bring sadness or sorrow. There's nothing one-dimensional when it comes to emotions, so it's important to understand that you can experience Jeong in complex ways. Jeong is part of all relationships in Korean culture, as well as Korean American culture. However, it can also refer to all relationships, and not just with people. Jeong can also apply to places, possessions, and animals. For instance, you can have a relationship with your hometown, birthplace, or country of origin. You can also have a relationship with a precious gift you received as a child, like your favorite stuffed animal or blanket, or even have Jeong with a workplace or organization. We all feel Jeong (love) with our pets, and as a therapist, I have treated many clients who grieved over the loss of their beloved pets and I've experienced this too.

Jeong comes naturally and develops over time, but it doesn't necessarily have to be a long period of time. In fact, it can be just as dynamic experiencing Jeong with someone or something you just met or encountered. Here's a perfect example. When you meet fellow K-Drama lovers or K-Pop stans, you feel an immediate Jeong and can start talking to them more than perhaps with your own family because of this kinship through the love of K-Dramas and K-Pop. There's an instant kismet of sorts because of the shared interest and experiences. All of us on my inaugural tours last year felt Jeong from the instant we met in the hotel lobby the first day, without having known one another before, because we were bonded over a K-Drama tour experience.

I'm often asked, "What's so great about K-Dramas?" I'm reminded of what one of my inaugural tour participants, a Venezuelan currently living in Canada, said about K-Dramas: "I love seeing how people-oriented Koreans are. I wish Venezuelans were like this and could learn from the Korean culture." She's describing Jeong. In the end, as mental health experts will tell you, we are connective and collective creatures.

My Favorite Examples of Jeong in K-Dramas:
- *Crash Landing on You*: Captain Ri's troop and Yoon Seri
- *My Mister*: Park Dong Hoon and Lee Jian
- *My Mister*: Lee Jian and Saman E&C
- *Navillera*: Shim Deok Cheol and Lee Chae Rok
- *Hometown Cha-Cha-Cha*: Gongjin and its townspeople
- *Reply 1988*: Ssangmun-dong parents and their kids
- *Start-Up*: Dalmi's halmuni and Han Ji Pyeong
- *Hospital Playlist*: The five doctor besties
- *Twenty-Five Twenty-One*: Na Heedo and Ko Yurim

My Mister, 2018

Here we are in the grand finale of my book, and as of this writing, I am thrilled to see that *Extraordinary Attorney Woo* and *Reborn Rich* have been nominated for International Emmy Awards. They're not the first K-Dramas to be nominated, but it still excites me when I see K-Dramas receiving accolades because that's a recent phenomenon, less than five years old. What validates me most in doing the work I do with K-Dramas is hearing stories from my followers and clients who resonate with my content. I also feel validated when I get recognized for this work and interviewed by media outlets. As a former journalist, I know that news is news, and it means I am making news in my own way. I'll never forget the moment I decided to take the leap to create Noona's Noonchi and then integrate K-Dramas into my clinical work. I didn't question it once I decided to do it because I thought (and still think), "K-Dramas help me with my mental health, so of course they can help others."

I'd like to highlight my favorite K-Drama again. *My Mister* has been my number one, while a close second is *Reply 1988*. My mental health deep dives come mainly from a professional lens, a mental health perspective where I also look at the impact of the K-Drama on my global community. One of my favorite things about *My Mister* is that talking about this K-Drama brings the Jeong with Koreans in Korea. This is very important to me. At the heart of my identity, I am Korean. I was born in Seoul, South Korea, and my parents chose to immigrate to the United States in 1974 when I was only several months old. However, they raised me as traditional Korean parents with what they knew of the Korea they had left. The main difference is that I was raised in a Western environment speaking English. Hence the cultural conflict and the complexities surrounding my bicultural identity that I outlined earlier. *My Mister* was my way of connecting on a deeper level with Koreans living in Korea. Based on my own research throughout 2022–2023, I found that *My Mister* was also a Korean fan favorite. This makes me so happy. As a family therapist, I look for patterns of behavior in families and communities. Also, finding similarities among people enhances belongingness, which is crucial to our mental health.

The fact that *My Mister* is both a favorite among Koreans and popular among foreigners is a huge piece of data that I am continuing to break down even as I write this book. Perhaps it's because I'm Korean American that I look for these facts. Sharing about *My Mister* has been a wonderful way to build relationships and make new friends in Korea. I have found that this K-Drama resonates with all ages. And it's my leverage in elevating the Jeong between my two cultures.

As *Forbes* writer Joan MacDonald puts it, "*My Mister* starts out grim, but by the end you feel better about yourself and other people." This is certainly true for me and what I have heard from others who've shared their first-hand experiences with this K-Drama.

To those who ask me, "What's your favorite K-Drama?" I explain it's *My Mister* because it transformed me. It made me introspective, and humbled me to see poignant acts of kindness and goodness. Others have their own experience with this K-Drama, and the conversations about *My Mister* appear to be endless. I love what my pal Chil Kong, a Nickelodeon consulting producer who calls himself a "rabid K-Drama fan" says about the show: "It's a story about how one simple of act of kindness (as the saying goes) is what transforms a young lady's hardened heart, which changes her life." The simple act of kindness that Chil is referring to is when the male protagonist, Park Dong Hoon (whom I talked about in Chapter 10, on life stages), asks the female protagonist, Lee Jian, to join the team dinner. Jian later shares that it was the first time anyone in the office took notice of her and how much she appreciated it. Although she hesitated, she did attend that team dinner and it started her journey of transformation.

As I've said before, this is a K-Drama I recommend to folks who are struggling with depression or feeling down, because they get to watch characters navigate their season of life where their change is quite evident by the K-Drama's end. We first meet them in their most downtrodden and discouraged state, and throughout the show, as the story progresses, we see a gradual but definitive growth, which therapists like to see. By the end of *My Mister* we are witnessing characters transformed, filled with hope, believing in their happiness, experiencing the beauty of humanity. This is helpful for any person to see, but especially for those who are experiencing depression or feeling depressed. Your mood slowly but surely improves, which is a realistic example of improvement in real life. There's a reconciliation of sorts that happens in the characters, particularly Jian, and that makes us feel good. The character transformation of Jian, as well as the real-life transformations of people I have met, explains the title of this book. I tell my clients that one small, positive change in your life is really all I ask for. In therapy, we talk about how one small change can lead to a large, systemic change, which can radically change your life for the better.

Because those who are familiar with my work know this is my favorite K-Drama, they try to watch it. Some have struggled watching it and some can't get through it. That is fine. Just because I believe a K-Drama benefits mental health does not mean it will specifically benefit yours.

In fact, my K-Drama lists are recommendations. They're optional. My lists are not something you must follow just because a therapist told you to. Mental health is not a linear process, and everyone is on their own journey when it comes to their mental health. Thus, what I suggest is simply what I suggest. I would not be an effective clinician if I recommended a K-Drama and it made you feel worse.

The disclaimer here is that I can do my best to make recommendations or suggestions for you based on my clinical expertise. I think long and hard about my lists, sometimes agonizing over them to ensure I am doing my best for my clients, followers, and colleagues.

Transformative Change

K-Dramas can be transforming. They can bring about a dramatic or radical change in one's character, behavior, nature, and perspective. It's why I love *My Mister* so much, because the transformation of Lee Jian was beautifully laid out and modeled for us the splendor of transformation. It inspires us to seek changes needed in our life for health and happiness. Although transformation is what provides us with the meaning and purpose for our mental health's sake, change is the key word here. It's why I do what I do. It's why I recommend K-Dramas as a tool to help you with your mental health. Change is what I look for since it's why you're coming to see me in the first place. I'm refraining from saying "good" change, since that simplifies things too much. What may be positive or good change for one person may not make sense for another person.

In family systems theory, which is the foundation of my work, there are two types of change we family therapists outline in our sessions. First-order change is a simple behavioral change, which can be reversible. It's doing more or less of something we are already doing. Meanwhile, second-order change—the kind we look for—is deciding to do something completely unknown or different than done before, fundamentally shifting one's perspective or line of thinking. Second-order change is a transformative, more permanent change in one's life. Through the lens of *My Mister*, an example of first-order change is when Jian decides to attend the team dinner she was invited to by Park Dong Hoon. This helps her get to know him (for various reasons in the plot), which turns into a friendship that softens her heart. Second-order change is when she decides to testify on his behalf (you'll have to watch to know what I mean) to save his job, regardless of what happens to her. She's willing to do anything she can to defend his character in front of executives. She puts herself on the line for his sake because she acknowledges he's changed her life with his kindness.

That, my friends, is transformation, which I hope you have gathered throughout the book. The 1992 K-Drama *Jil-tu* transformed the relationship I had to my culture, my country of origin. From that summer on, the second-order change for me was choosing to lean into my culture for the sake of my emotional, social, and psychological well-being. Everything we're talking about in my session, on my platform, in my workshops, and on my tours is about what K-Dramas have done to bring impactful, transformative change in our lives. I'd like to end by sharing the story of my son's discovery of the meaning surrounding Jeong.

When my son (the third child) was applying to college, he decided to write his common application essay on *Reply 1988* and Jeong.

Of course, you can imagine how thrilled I was. I hadn't realized until reading his essay that he understood Jeong, but clearly he grasped the emotionality behind it through *Reply 1988*. What touched me was how my son connected the dots between the Jeong he witnessed in the K-Drama among the family and friends to his grandparents. *Reply 1988* happened to be my parents' first and last K-Drama, as of this writing. Believe it or not, they don't watch K-Dramas, but they decided to watch *Reply 1988* with their grandchildren over Thanksgiving a few years ago. My son talked about his grandfather feeling nostalgic watching *Reply 1988* because he got to live out those years through the K-Drama and learn what Korea looked like at the time. My parents immigrated with me to the United States in 1974 so they missed out on life in Korea since then. They don't know what it looked like except through *Reply 1988*. My son pointed out the Jeong he realized my father was experiencing via the K-Drama to a life he didn't experience in Korea during those years.

After my son's high school graduation in the summer of 2022, we went to Korea for the first time in 10 years, but without my older two kids because they were adulting. It was a wonderful trip, and on the day before we were slated to head back home, I took my boys to one of the largest food markets, Gwangjang Market. We ate lunch at one of the stands and on our ride in the taxi, my son (who wrote the college essay on *Reply 1988*) told me he saw Jeong from the halmunis (grandmothers) they were sitting next to in the booth who slid over ever so discreetly to make room for my boys when there really wasn't room.

They also noticed my sons didn't have napkins and handed some to them. I was distracted but I recall noticing their behavior without thinking twice about it. However, my son said, "That was so nice, like the halmunis in the K-Dramas." I hadn't realized that, through watching K-Dramas, whether with us or on his own, my son was making meaning in his own life at 18 years old (at the time). There was such poignancy in his words and sure, he's Korean American so there's the Jeong innate in our Korean culture that perhaps he picks up on. However, based on his college essay, and the fact that, aside from K-Dramas and the food, our kids didn't have too much exposure to traditional Korean culture, I found that he learned about Jeong by the behavior he watched onscreen.

My Transformation

"I analyze K-Dramas for a living."

This has become my catchphrase when I meet new people who ask what I do. It sure does grab their attention! They lean in to find out more because they're curious, or they get so excited and jump at the chance to get to know me. In recent months (as of this writing), I am finding the latter happening more often because half the time I meet someone new, they're already a K-Drama fan. I am beginning to take ownership of this phrase because it's true. In some sense, I joke with others that I manifested it out of my love of K-Dramas. A majority of my workshops in the last year included K-Dramas for mental health, regardless of the audience. Just a few years ago, I would have discussed with the organizational client about including K-Dramas, but now when they ask me to speak on a specific topic, I indicate I'll also be including K-Drama examples on those topics. The response has been encouraging. What started out as a joke, "I analyze K-Dramas for a living," is what has transformed me. In turn, it has transformed my clinical practice. I am a better clinician today because of K-Dramas and how they benefit my mental health. It doesn't mean I am always happy or even healthy. (Remember what I said about mental health not being linear.) It means that K-Dramas teach me ways to improve my emotional, social, and psychological well-being. The wisdom from the K-Drama characters hasn't ceased to amaze me when I see how it changes my own behavior, especially when it comes to my own family. Yes, I'm analyzing K-Dramas for a living, but the "living" I'm talking about is pursuing a life you want to live for healing and happiness.

K-Dramas have been my form of self-care for years. Bringing them into my work because I was so confident about how they helped me has been so natural. I think that's why I came to build my own Noona's Noonchi community. It came out of authenticity, my personal passion. As a clinician, I feel most validated when people tell me they see how I truly believe in what I am telling them about K-Dramas for mental health, but also what I have observed using my "noonchi" when it comes to mental health among all generations. Clients see me as the expert and it's important for the therapeutic relationship, not just in therapy sessions but also in my workshops, for what I am sharing to resonate with the audience, my community. I need them to see my authenticity and vulnerability, or I feel that I am not making an impact. I hadn't realized my own impact until I launched my global K-Culture tours.

I am practicing what I teach here by recognizing my own accomplishments and success, which is difficult as an Asian American. When I saw folks on that tour bus discussing that they had signed up as quickly as they could when they heard about my tours, I realized that I do have my own global community at Noona's Noonchi. I keep downplaying it because when you're in the social media influencer space, you tend to compare yourself with others by the number of followers you have. In that sense, I do not feel I have an online presence as strong as others might. However, people have pointed out to me how my online presence has powerfully translated to my business and clinical practice. Many of my clients have told me how thankful they are for Noona's Noonchi, and that they hope I know the impact I am making. Hearing this is what validates me the most as a clinician, speaker, and coach. I now have a global company, Noona's Noonchi, LLC (in the United States) and Noona's Noonchi, Inc. (based in South Korea). I do, after all, analyze K-Dramas for a living.

How can K-Dramas transform your life? If you're watching them, they already are, because you're reflecting on the stories, making meaning behind what you're feeling, thinking, and seeking impactful change in your life for healing. If you are thinking about watching K-Dramas for the sake of your mental health, I hope my book is a catalyst for you to embark on a healing journey of introspection to seek transformation in a unique and fun way. If K-Dramas have transformed my life, and transformed that of my ever-growing community, I believe they can transform yours.

Resource List

My Top 20 Favorite K-Dramas of All Time

Listed in descending order, with the last being the most favorite. Special recognition also goes to 1992's *Jealousy*. It was my very first K-Drama and it changed my life.

20. *Full House*
19. *Coffee Prince*
18. *Secret Garden*
17. *My Lovely Sam Soon*
16. *When the Camellia Blooms*
15. *Hospital Playlist*
14. *My Liberation Notes*
13. *The Red Sleeve*
12. *Crash Landing on You*
11. *Our Blues*
10. *I Hear Your Voice*
9. *Goblin*
8. *Healer*
7. *Extraordinary Attorney Woo*
6. *Master's Sun*
5. *Hometown Cha-Cha-Cha*

4. *Mr. Sunshine*
3. *The Greatest Love*
2. *Reply 1988*
1. *My Mister*

References

Clayton, Anita, MD, and Phillip T. Ninan, MD. "Depression or Menopause? Presentation and Management of Major Depressive Disorder in Perimenopausal and Postmenopausal Women." *Primary Care Companion, Journal of Clinical Psychiatry* 12, no. 1 (2010). https://www.ncbi.nlm.nih.gov/pmc/articles/PMC2882 813/#:~:text=Women%20in%20the%20menopausal%20 transition%20are%20at%20increased,major%20depressive% 20disorder%20(MDD).&text=Routine%20screening%20for %20MDD%20and,is%20crucial%20for%20effective%20 management.&text=Potential%20interventions%20include%20 estrogen%20therapy%2C%20antidepressant%20medicati ons%2C%20or%20both.

"Global Tourism Market Trends on Track to Recovery (data)." Invest Korea, 2022. https://www.investkorea.org/ik-en/cntnts/i-322/ web.do.

Hae-rin, Lee. "Korea aims to curtail suicide rate with more frequent mental health checkups." *Korea Times,* April 14, 2023. https://www. koreatimes.co.kr/www/nation/2023/08/113_349065.html.

Jae-hee, Choi. "We need more 'Attorney Woos,' says Florida's first publicly autistic attorney." *Korea Herald,* July 20, 2022. https:// www.koreaherald.com/view.php?ud=20220720000804.

Kim, Charles R. *Beyond Death: The Politics of Suicide and Martyrdom in Korea.* University of Washington Center for Korea Studies, 2019.

Kim, Regina, "The K-Drama Renaissance: How South Korean Entertainment Took Over Your TV." *Elle,* August 17, 2021. https://www.elle.com/culture/movies-tv/a37293494/korean-drama-renaissance-explained/.

Linehan, Marsha M. "The Course and Evolution of Dialectical Behavior Therapy." *American Journal of Psychotherapy* 69, no. 2 (2015): 97–110. Published online April 30, 2018. https://psychotherapy.psychiatryonline.org/doi/10.1176/appi.psychotherapy.2015.69.2.97.

Littleton, Cynthia, and Sara Layne. "K-Dramas Can't Be Denied: Global Streaming Spurs Demand for Asian Content Platforms." *Variety,* August 18, 2022. https://variety.com/2022/streaming/news/korean-dramas-kocowa-viki-asiancrush-kcon-1235344275/.

Marcin, Ashley. "9 Ways Crying May Benefit Your Health." *Healthline,* April 14, 2017. https://www.healthline.com/health/benefits-of-crying#mood https://www.linkedin.com/in/elliemidds/?src=or-search&veh=www.google.com%257Cor-search.

Olivine, Ashley, PhD, MPH. "The Meaning of Escapism in Psychology." VeryWellHealth.com. https://www.verywellhealth.com/escapism-7565008#:~:text=Any%20life%20change%20can%20lead,increase%20the%20desire%20to%20escape.

Rappeneau, Virginie, and Anne Berod, "Reconsidering Depression as a Risk Factor for Substance Use Disorder: Insights from Rodent Models." *Neuroscience & Biobehavioral Reviews* 77 (June 2017) 303–316. https://pubmed.ncbi.nlm.nih.gov/28385601/.

Veale, Jennifer. "South Koreans Are Shaken by a Celebrity Suicide." *Time,* October 6, 2008. https://content.time.com/time/world/article/0,8599,1847437,00.html.

Waldinger, Robert. "What makes a good life? Lessons from the longest study on happiness." TED Talk, YouTube, January 25, 2016. https://youtu.be/8KkKuTCFvzI?si=9podbhWhxxidPREu.

Yehuda, Rachel, and Amy Lehrner. "Intergenerational Transmission of Trauma Effects: Putative Role of Epigenetic Mechanisms." *World Psychiatry* 17, no. 3 (October 2018): 243–257. Published online September 7, 2018. https://www.ncbi.nlm.nih.gov/pmc/arti cles/PMC6127768/#:~:text=The%20concept%20of%20inter generational%20trauma%20was%20introduced%20in%20the%20 psychiatric,offspring%20of%20Holocaust%20survivors8.

Yeon-soo, Kwak. "Popularity of K-content drives boom in Korean language learning," *Korea Times,* March 16, 2022. https://www. koreatimes.co.kr/www/culture/2022/03/199_325603.html.

Yeon-soo, Kwak. "Remake boom of K-dramas is a testament to their brilliant storytelling." *Korea Times,* June 3, 2021. https://www. koreatimes.co.kr/www/art/2023/06/398_309849.html.

Yeung, Jesse. "South Korea brought K-pop and K-dramas to the world. The Korean language could be next." CNN, January 7, 2023. https:// edition.cnn.com/2023/01/17/asia/korean-language-learning-rise-hallyu-intl-hnk-dst/index.html#:~:text=There's%20never%20 been%20a%20better,call%20the%20%E2%80%9CKorean%20 wave.%E2%80%9D.

Young-sil, Yoon. "Korea Cultural Wave Puts Korea 7th in World Cultural Power." *Business Korea,* July 11, 2023. https://www.busi nesskorea.co.kr/news/articleView.html?idxno=118177.

Acknowledgments

Thank you so much to Wiley Publishing for giving me this chance of a lifetime. I'm especially grateful to Victoria Savanh, Wiley's acquisitions editor, for believing in my work. And another special thank you to Neva Talladen, my developmental editor, for her patience and encouragement throughout the book writing process!

Thank you so much to those who agreed to be interviewed for my book. Thank you for sharing your time and stories.

A special thank you to my inaugural K-Drama tour groups of 2023, who inspired me at the very end of writing this book, when things got tough. What a privilege it is to meet my followers in person and travel to K-Drama sites together around South Korea. You encouraged me so much more than you know.

Finally, thank you so much to my Noona's Noonchi global community, for the belongingness. Without your constant engagement and support online, this book would not have been possible.

About the Author

Jeanie is a second-generation Korean American licensed clinician, speaker, executive coach, and published author. She is a Licensed Marriage and Family Therapist with specialized training as a Certified Clinical Trauma Professional and in Mindfulness-Based Stress Reduction (MBSR). Her expertise includes grief, trauma, intergenerational mental health, workplace mental health, and K-Dramas for mental health. She followed a calling in the field after a diverse career path, starting as a broadcast journalist in Washington, DC, in the 1990s, then attending business school.

Jeanie is the founder of Noona's Noonchi®, Inc., a global wellness and tourism company created out of her social media influence as Noona's Noonchi—a clinician, speaker, and coach who deep dives into K-Dramas from a mental health perspective. Jeanie serves as a subject matter expert on mental health for media outlets around the world. She is also the founder and CEO of Your Change Provider, PLLC®, a clinical practice based in the United States, founded on her unique, trademarked framework titled Cultural Confidence®, providing psychoeducation across all sectors, most notably with Google, H&M, J. Crew, Microsoft, Medtronic, and the NFL. She has also spearheaded her program for national Asian nonprofits, including the Asian American Journalists Association (AAJA), the Council of Korean Americans (CKA), the Society of Asian Scientists and Engineers (SASE), and the National Association of Asian American Professionals (NAAAP).

She is an active volunteer in the AAPI community, serving as board chair of Asian Mental Health Collective (AMHC), and is a facilitator for the Council of Korean Americans' Network of Korean American Leaders (NetKAL) program. In 2019, Jeanie created the Self-Care & Wellness program for NAAAP, and founded her own nonprofit organization in 2020, Authentic Self-Care & Wellness, Inc.

Jeanie is most proud of her family. She's been married to her husband since 1998. Together they have four children.

Index

Note: Page numbers in *italics* indicate figures and tables.